Living with ObamaCare

Living with ObamaCare

A Consumer's Guide

John C. Goodman

About the Author

John C. Goodman is president and CEO of the National Center for Policy Analysis, an independent research institute, where he is the Kellye Wright Fellow in Health Care. Widely known as the "father of health savings accounts," Goodman has written numerous popular and scholarly articles on health reform and has authored 12 books. He received a Ph.D. in economics from Columbia University and taught at several universities before founding the NCPA in 1983.

Other books by the author:

Priceless: Curing the Healthcare Crisis (Oakland, Calif.: Independent Institute, 2012).

Handbook on State Health Care Reform, with Michael Bond, Devon M. Herrick, Gerald L. Musgrave, Pamela Villarreal and Joe Barnett (Dallas, Texas: National Center for Policy Analysis, 2007).

Leaving Women Behind: Modern Families, Outdated Laws, with Kimberley A. Strassel and Celeste Colgan (Lanham, Md.: Rowman and Littlefield, 2005).

Lives at Risk: Single Payer National Health Insurance Around the World, with Gerald Musgrave and Devon M. Herrick (Lanham, Md.: Rowman and Littlefield, 2004).

Economics of Public Policy, 5th ed., with Edwin Dolan (St. Paul, Minn.: West Publishing Co., 1995).

Patient Power: Solving America's Health Care Crisis (Washington, D.C.: Cato Institute, 1992).

Voluntary Welfare; A Greater Role for Private Charities (Sidney, Australia: Centre for Independent Studies, 1990).

Fighting the War of Ideas in Latin America (Dallas, Texas: National Center for Policy Analysis, 1989).

Privatization (Dallas, Texas: National Center for Policy Analysis, 1985).

Social Security in the United Kingdom: Contracting Out of the System (Washington, D.C.: American Enterprise Institute, 1981).

National Health Care in Great Britain: Lessons for the U.S.A. (Dallas, Texas: Fisher Institute, 1980).

The Regulation of Medical Care: Is the Price Too High? (San Francisco, Calif.: Cato Institute, 1980).

National Center for Policy Analysis

14180 Dallas Parkway, Ste. 350

Dallas, Texas 75254

www.ncpa.org

ISBN 978-1-56808-234-9

Printed in the United States of America.

Table of Contents

Introduction: Why You Need This Book

The goal of the Affordable Care Act (what many people call ObamaCare) is to completely remake the nation's health care system. It is the most revolutionary public policy reform since the War on Poverty in the 1960s, with many laudable goals. But the methods are controversial. Further, this reform occurred at a time when the nation's capital is more polarized along partisan lines than at any time in recent history. As a result, no one is telling you the whole truth. Every revolutionary change produces winners and losers. There is some good and some bad. That's true of all change. But you would never know that in this highly politicized atmosphere.

All we hear from the White House and congressional Democrats are the benefits of change. When they appear on TV news shows, armed with talking points — they promptly list every good thing about the reform they can think of. For the past three years, they have sold ObamaCare the way Madison Avenue sells soap.

But the Republicans are just as bad, in the opposite way. Watch an interview on TV, and you will hear everything bad about the reform they can think of. Conservatives are trying to convince you that ObamaCare is a disaster in the same way Madison Avenue tries to get you to quit smoking or lose weight.

In this partisan environment, you simply cannot get objective information about what health reform means for you, at least not from anyone in Washington, D.C.

No matter what happens — problems with the exchange website, insurance policies canceled, new insurance deductibles shockingly higher, networks of doctors surprisingly narrower — politicians will only give you spin. No one in Washington has the slightest interest in helping you understand the objective facts.

Where else might you turn? Insurance companies? Essentially, they will carry out health care reform. They are going to run virtually every aspect of it. And for the past three years they have been planning everything — what premiums they will charge, how high the deductibles will be, which doctors and hospitals will be in their networks—they have been studying and thinking intensively about everything involved in health reform

But when was the last time you saw the CEO of a health insurance company on a TV news show answering questions? You probably can't name a single example. Do you know how unusual that is? This country is about to experience the most revolutionary change in public policy in 50 years, yet you never see the people who are going to actually facilitate that change on TV answering questions posed by …. well … by anybody!

Why aren't the insurance executives trying to help us understand what is going on? The short answer to that question is that the insurance companies have been cowed. They are afraid of the White House, afraid of the Democrats and afraid of the Republicans as well. So they are not saying anything.

What about the news media? Sadly, they haven't done their job either. Little has happened in the past three months that wasn't predicted over three years ago. The Congressional Budget Office, the Medicare chief actuary, the Medicare Trustees Report — you could have gone to several good and respected sources to anticipate what is happening right now, both good and bad. But almost none of this made its way into the daily newspapers. The reason? Reporters were too busy reporting the inside-the-Beltway spin.

This book was written to fill a vacuum. You need an objective, unbiased look at health reform, and we believe this book will give you that perspective.

Let me know if we have met your needs by leaving a comment or question at FreeOurHealthCareNow.org.

John C. Goodman

P.S. This book was made possible through the tireless efforts of the staff of the National Center for Policy Analysis. Special thanks go to Devon Herrick, Joe Barnett, Courtney MacDonell, Jake Casey and David Weisser.

Off to a Rocky Start

The Affordable Care Act (ACA) is built on five primary pillars:

1) An individual mandate that requires most people to have health insurance;
2) An employer mandate requiring employer coverage for most employees;
3) Health insurance exchanges where individuals can easily obtain coverage regardless of health status;
4) Generous income-based subsidies to assist those who otherwise could not afford health coverage; and
5) Medicaid for those with low incomes.

Advocates of health reform worry that without the proper functioning of all five of these pillars, reform will not achieve its goal of universal coverage that is affordable. They have reason to worry. Various factors have weakened all five.

The first pillar weakened in June 2012, when the U.S. Supreme Court ruled that states could not be forced to expand their Medicaid programs. Many states have decided the costs of expansion outweigh the benefits. As a result, millions of people below the federal poverty level will not have access to Medicaid, or to subsidized private insurance in the exchanges.

The second pillar — the requirement that employers must cover their employees — also weakened when the Obama administration postponed implementation for up to two years. Further, the administration has ruled that the individual mandate will be temporarily suspended for anyone who lost insurance through no fault of his or her own (a number expected to reach more than 15 million by the end of 2014), and insiders are predicting that the mandate may be suspended for everyone — at least for this year.

The third pillar — rollout of the exchanges — has also not gone as intended. The 37 exchanges operated by the federal government were not ready on time. With a few notable exceptions, the state exchanges didn't fare much better.

The fourth pillar is subject to "sticker shock." As people enter the exchanges, they are finding that even with subsidies, the premiums for plans that give them access to the same doctors they previously saw are higher than anyone expected. The fifth pillar is Medicaid, whose health care providers will be overwhelmed by new enrollees.

Cancellations and Delays. A mid-September 2013 report identified 19 separate delays involving provisions in the Affordable Care Act,[1] and quite a few more have appeared since. Here are a few of the most important:

- As noted, the employer mandate due to take effect in 2014 has been delayed until 2016 for employees with 50 to 99 fulltime employees, and to 2015 for larger employers.
- The small-business insurance exchange has also been pushed back a year.
- A popular consumer protection, the limit on out-of-pocket spending, was delayed one year for some group health plans.[2]
- The long-term-care insurance program (referred to as the CLASS ACT) was canceled altogether when it was determined the program would be unsustainable.[3]
- As noted, the individual mandate has been waived for people whose plans have been recently canceled.[4]
- There were several changes in the deadline people must meet to sign up for insurance that became effective on January 1, 2014.
- Another change allows people whose plans were recently canceled to purchase a low-cost catastrophic plan that doesn't comply with the required benefits package.

Arguably, the worst delay of all involved the failure of the health insurance exchanges to be ready on time. Technical glitches continue to plague the federal and state websites that were supposed to offer one-stop shopping for health coverage.

A Computer System That Isn't Working Very Well. The process was supposed to work like this: You enter a few bits of information about yourself into a website. The system then connects to the Internal Revenue Service (IRS), pulls up your most recent tax return and calculates your "modified gross income," something most people won't be able to do on their own. Next, the system contacts the Social Security Administration to find out many different employers you have. It then goes to the Labor Department to see if any of those employers have offered you "affordable insurance," a term most people won't be able to define on their own. Finally, the system connects to your state's Medicaid program to see if you are eligible for Medicaid, yet another determination most people won't be able to make on their own. And along the way the system will likely ask you additional questions and require additional input.

If the system determines you are eligible to enter a health insurance exchange, it then tells you what your subsidy will be, gives you choices among an array of private health plans available in your area and offers you the opportunity to enroll in one of them. For each option, you learn what premium you will have to pay, what deductibles and copayments you will face and which doctors and hospitals are in the plan's network.

All of this was supposed to happen in about seven minutes.

Except that none of this is actually working the way it is supposed to. The Department of Health and Human Services has a computer system that seems unable to talk to most other government agencies. As a result, it is unable to verify how much you earn or who your employer is or whether the insurance your employer offers is "compliant" and "affordable." And to overcome these difficulties, the system has been effectively jury-rigged.

Now the system asks you to guess what your income will be this year — not your "modified gross income," the real number the system needs, just "income." This guarantees that whatever number people enter is almost certainly going to be wrong. As a result, at tax time next year, your tax preparer will have to figure out if last year's subsidy was too high or too low, in which case you will owe more in taxes or you will be entitled to a bigger refund.

When entering an income estimate, people will be on their honor to be truthful — which is a problem, because people are discovering that the lower the number they report, the bigger their subsidy.

3

Also, if people get a larger subsidy than the one they are entitled to, government's ability to reclaim the overpayment is limited. So people have a perverse incentive to under-report their income.

None of this will become an issue, however, if people are unable to actually purchase insurance online, and that appears to be the case for millions of people.[5]

- A Florida man tried to enroll more than 100 times before he was successful; at the time of this writing, he has still been unable to make his first premium payment.
- A teacher in Michigan claimed the government's website has been unable to verify her identity for six weeks — she worked withboththecomputerandthegovernment'stelephonehotline.
- A Pennsylvania man finally enrolled (after two months of effort) and was told by the government website that his cost sharing was limited to $175; however, his insurer now tells him that the actual amount is 20 times that high.
- A Colorado man used his dog's name as a password security question; the system enrolled the dog, but he was unable to enroll himself.
- When Senator Rand Paul (R-Ky.) tried to enroll his family in a private health plan, the system enrolled his son in Medicaid instead.[6]
- According to an Associated Press investigation, even in early 2014, the ACA website would not allow you to add a baby to your health plan; it also couldn't handle marriages, divorces or even a move to another community.[7]

Many problems appear to have been fixed, but information technology experts claim the website fixes are superficial. Though the federal exchange website appears to be working for visitors, it is still having problems talking to the insurers.[8] By some estimates, one-fourth of the applications on HealthCare. gov have data errors. Health plans are not sure if the person they enrolled actually qualifies for subsidies or is even eligible to enroll. On January 1, 2014, the day that the new (ObamaCare) insurance first became effective, people began to learn what that means. For instance, at one Virginia hospital, dozens of patients who thought they were insured discovered that the hospital could not verify that fact. After being asked to pay for care out of pocket, many patients left without being treated. And a doctor's office in Chicago spent two hours on the phone trying to get authorization for surgery from an insurer and finally gave up.[9]

It appears that about 2 million people successfully enrolled in private insurance plans by January 1, 2014. But consumers are not actually covered until they've made their first premium payment, and third-party billing companies estimate that only about half of those enrolled have made that first payment.[10]

Initially, consumers were to have selected plans by December 15 and made their first payment by December 31 in order to have coverage by January 1. Missing these deadlines would mean coverage could not begin until February 1. To avoid gaps in coverage that could potentially leave millions of people temporarily uninsured and exposed to costly medical bills, the Obama administration moved the deadline for enrolling to December 23, with the first payment due by January 1. Then, the administration asked the health insurance industry to extend the payment deadline even further. The health insurance trade association announced insurers would accept payments as late as January 10 for coverage retroactive to January 1.[11]

Also, people who make the first month's premium payment may not make the second payment — and this is especially true of people who are not used to making monthly payments to insurance companies, and of people who live from paycheck to paycheck. We will probably not know until 2015 how many people were successfully insured in the first full year of health reform.

Then there is the issue of identity theft. To process applications, the exchange data hubs necessarily must have access to personal information, such as income, Social Security numbers, employer, home address and more — a veritable treasure trove of information identity thieves would love to get their hands on.[12] When banks, financial institutions and normal businesses create sites that process

5

financial transactions, the designers build site security into the original design. But according to a professional hacking expert who testified on Capitol Hill, this was not done with the government's health care website. Further, going back to retroactively make the system secure will take at least another year.[13]

Losing the Coverage That You Liked. Experts believe that as many as 6 million people saw their health insurance canceled in 2013 due to the ACA, and that number is expected to climb.[14] Health insurance expert Robert Laszewski estimates that the number losing their individual coverage will reach more than 15 million by the end of 2014.[15]

Defenders of the new law claim that most people losing their insurance are giving up skimpy coverage for much better benefits. But it is becoming increasingly apparent that isn't always the case. Take the case of Edie Sundby, a California woman who has a rare form of cancer that is almost always fatal.[16] She is alive thanks to the efforts of doctors in San Diego, at Stanford University and in Texas. Over the past year, UnitedHealthcare spent $1.2 million on Edie's medical expenses. But she has been informed that her insurance is being canceled, and she must now buy insurance in the new California exchange. Yet only one plan will allow her to continue seeing her San Diego doctors, and no plan will pay for the doctors at Stanford or in Texas.

There is a good chance the kind of coverage Edie Sundby had will never again be seen in the individual market in this country. The reason: Insurers now face a new set of perverse incentives. What insurance company wants a patient who needs $1.2 million worth of medical care?

Race to the Bottom.[17] Prior to the ACA, most insurers selling individual policies were allowed to charge individuals premiums that reflected their expected health care costs. This practice is similar to life insurance, casualty insurance or almost any other kind of insurance — except that in these other markets people don't lose their insurance whenever they switch jobs. In a normal insurance market, you expect to pay premiums that are actuarially fair. The

Affordable Care Act ended this. Instead, insurers are now required to practice community rating, under which the healthy and the sick within a given area will all be charged the same premium.

You don't even have to be in the business to understand what kind of incentives that creates for the insurers. If the healthy are overcharged so that the sick can be undercharged, insurance companies can expect to make profits on the healthy and face losses on the sick. This means that it is in the self-interest of every insurer to attract the healthy and avoid the sick.

How can they accomplish that? One way is to design plans that are attractive to the healthy but unattractive to the sick.

Under a typical California exchange plan, for example, patients will make only nominal copayments when they see a doctor, get a blood test or have an X-ray exam — activities that are often discretionary and the source of a great deal of unnecessary care. But if they go into a hospital (where patients have almost no control over what is done and usually know nothing about real costs), they will be charged from 10 to 20 percent of the bill, up to the maximum out-of-pocket limit. For an individual earning only a few thousand dollars above the poverty level in 2012, for instance, a hospital visit could cost $2,500 in out-of-pocket payments. For a lower-middle income patient, the charge would be $6,350. A moderate-income family could end up paying hospital expenses of $12,700 every year!

Clearly this plan will attract people who don't plan to enter a hospital and deter people for whom a hospital stay is likely.

Think of an insurance plan as having three main components: 1) a premium, 2) a list of covered benefits and 3) a network of doctors, hospitals and other providers. The Affordable Care Act strictly regulates all your benefits — contraceptives, mammograms and a lengthy set of preventive procedures, for example, are all free. At the same time, health plans have been given enormous freedom to set their own (community-rated) premiums and choose their own networks. They are using that freedom in yet another way to attract the healthy and avoid the sick.

Insurers apparently believe that only sick people (who plan to spend a lot of health care dollars) pay close attention to networks. Healthy people tend to buy on price. Thus, by keeping provider fees so low that only a minority of physicians will agree to treat the patients, some insurers are able to quote lower premiums. They are banking on attracting healthy customers, not customers who need medical care. [Note: Even after insurers do this, the community-rated premiums may still be surprisingly high. See, "How Much Will My Health Insurance Cost?"]

As a result, there is a race to the bottom on access — with private plans in the exchanges looking increasingly like Medicaid, just as many subsidized plans do in Massachusetts, the prototype for national reform.

Winners and Losers. Regulation creates winners and losers. In this book, we will identify quite a few groups that fall into each camp. The Affordable Care Act does this based on public policy goals. An example is the policy of community rating: charging people the same premium regardless of expected health care costs. Community rating will cause younger, healthier people to be charged more than their expected costs so that older, less healthy, individuals can pay less — and this happens even though older enrollees generally have higher incomes and more assets than younger enrollees.

In a typical insurance pool in an average year, about 5 percent of the enrollees will be responsible for about half of the health care costs. These are the enrollees who experience expensive medical problems. The other half is spent by the remaining 95 percent. Since a person's health is unpredictable, we don't always know which enrollee will fall into which group. But we can often say which people are more likely to be in the 5 percent.

The promise of health reform is that you cannot be charged a higher premium simply because you are likely to be in the 5 percent. The other side of that promise is that if you are basically healthy and expect to remain that way, you will pay a higher premium than you otherwise would have paid.

Many people were surprised to lose their private insurance coverage, and many more experienced sticker shock when they entered the exchanges. Why? Because the Obama administration has not been frank in alerting people about what to expect. For the past three years, the White House has talked only about the winners and how much they are expected to gain. Virtually nothing has been said about the losers and what they should expect to lose.

Overview: Major Features of Health Reform

Here are some of the most important features of the health reform law with delays and exemptions by the Obama administration.

Structural Features of Reform

- As of January 1, 2014, the law requires you to have health insurance and to attach proof of insurance to next year's tax return, unless you have a special exemption or a waiver.
- If you fail to enroll in a health plan by March 31, you will be fined. For individuals, the fine is $95 or 1 percent of income, whichever is greater, rising to $695 or 2.5 percent of income by 2016. For families, the penalty is $285 or 10 percent of household income, rising to $2,085 or 2.5 percent of income by 2016.
- If your company employs 50 or more workers and fails to offer health insurance, it may be fined as much as $2,000 per employee per year beginning in 2016. Large employers have until 2015 to offer coverage to at least 70 percent of their employees, or be fined.
- If you are not covered by an employer plan, Medicare, Medicaid or other government plan, you are probably entitled to buy insurance in a government-regulated health insurance exchange.

Some Major Benefits of the Reform. Some of the touted benefits of reform are not new. For example, since 1996, federal law has barred insurers from dropping your coverage just because you get sick — despite repeated attempts to make us believe otherwise. However, the following changes are new:

- You may be able to buy insurance you could not previously afford. Beginning in 2014, for example, a couple with an income of twice the poverty level (currently $31,020) will be able to buy insurance for an annual premium no higher than 6.3 percent of their income ($1,954).
- If you have a pre-existing condition, you will be able to buy insurance for the same premium as that paid by people in good health.
- If you have an expensive and ongoing health problem, there will be no lifetime limits on your health insurance coverage.
- The Congressional Budget Office (CBO) expects that after health reform is fully implemented (2022), 25 million otherwise uninsured people will obtain health insurance. However, 30 million will still be uninsured.[18]

Some Major Costs of the Reform. In general, for every benefit, there is an offsetting cost. But more than half the costs of this reform will be borne by the elderly and disabled on Medicare:

- $716 billion of health reform's 10-year cost (2013-2022) will be paid for by cuts in spending on Medicare enrollees, according to the Congressional Budget Office.[19]
- In addition, new taxes have been placed on drugs and on such medical devices as wheelchairs, crutches, pacemakers, artificial joints and so on — items largely used by Medicare enrollees.

Reduced spending and reduced subsidies will have an especially big impact on seniors:

- Of the 15 million people expected to enroll in Medicare Advantage programs, 7.5 million will lose their plans entirely, according to Medicare's chief actuary, and the remainder will face higher premiums and lower benefits.[20]
- Nearly 6 million retired employees will lose their employer drug coverage, according to the 2010 Medicare Trustees report.

And other measures will affect the general population:

- A new tax on health insurance is likely to cost the families of employees of small businesses more than $500 a year in higher premiums.[21]
- A 40 percent tax on the extra coverage provided by expensive "Cadillac" plans will apply to about one-third of all private health insurance plans by 2019, and because the tax threshold is not indexed to medical inflation, over time the tax will eventually reach every health plan.
- Scores of other items will be taxed, ranging from tanning salons to the sale of your home, in some cases.

Some benefits have hidden costs:

- Health insurers are raising premiums for everyone in order to charge people with pre-existing conditions less than the expected cost of their care. Some young people, for example, have seen a doubling or tripling of their premiums.[22]
- Insurers are also trying to cover the higher costs of sicker enrollees with higher deductibles and narrow networks that cover only some of the doctors and hospitals in areas where people live.
- In order for employers to provide health insurance (or more generous insurance) to their employees, they will have to reduce what they pay in wages and in other benefits.
- The CBO estimates that 800,000 fewer people will be employed as a result of the health care law because of the higher cost of labor for employers, and that the number could eventually exceed 1 million.[23]

What Health Reform Does Not Do. During the debate leading up to health reform legislation, participants discussed the many problems we face as a nation along with the goals of reform. Here are some goals that will not be achieved:

Health care costs will probably rise rather than fall. Although the CBO initially predicted a slight lowering of overall health care costs in future years, it is now expressing doubts.[24] An analysis by the Office of the Medicare Actuary predicts that the new law will increase rather than decrease health care spending.[25] The graph below shows the prediction of the RAND Corporation, a respected private think tank.[26] And one of the architects of the reform's design, Massachusetts Institute of Technology economist Jonathan Gruber, finally admitted that nothing will lower health care spending.[27]

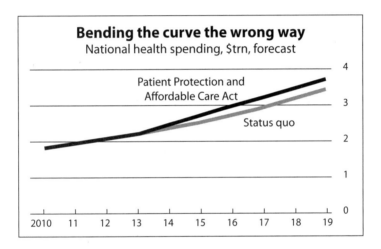

Source: RAND Corporation

Fortunately, the rate of increase in health care spending has been falling for the past decade and has been well below the historical trend since 2009. If this trend continues the reform will be less costly than originally estimated. This favorable development, however, began before the new health reform law was passed and it seems unrelated to any of its provisions.[28]

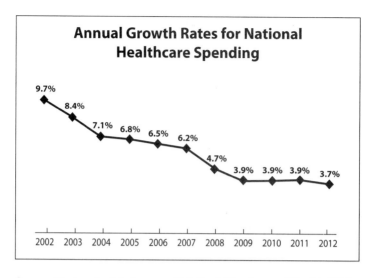

Source: *Centers for Medicare and Medicaid Services and* Health Affairs

Despite promises that the elderly and the disabled would gain from the reform, Medicare insurance is likely to radically change. A report from Medicare's actuaries explains:[29]

- Medicare fees paid to doctors and hospitals will fall below Medicaid levels by 2019, and going forward, they will fall increasingly behind the rates paid by other insurers.

- By 2050, Medicare fees are projected to be only one-half of what the private sector pays.

- By 2080, they will be only one-third.

Harvard University health economist Joe Newhouse explains what will happen if we follow this projected path. Seniors and the disabled will have increasingly less access to care, as providers turn first to the better-paying patients. In the near future, the fate of Medicare patients might come to resemble that of today's Medicaid enrollees, or even worse — the elderly and the disabled may have to seek care at community health centers and the emergency rooms of safety net hospitals.[30]

Will future Congresses and future presidents actually allow this to happen? Both President Obama and Congress have committedtoit.Butotheractionssuggestthattheircommitment may be weak. For example, current federal law is supposed to limit Medicare fee increases to doctors to no more than the rate of growth of national income. But for the past seven years, Congress stepped in on 14 occasions to prevent these limits from being imposed.[31]

Health insurance will not be portable for most people. The vast majority of people with private health insurance will continue to get job-based insurance. This means that when you leave your job, you will lose your coverage and be forced to find new insurance elsewhere.

People with the same incomes will not be treated the same way under the tax law. One of the complaints about the pre-ObamaCare system is that it was unfair — treating people differently depending on their income and where they obtained their health coverage. In fact, the after-tax cost of health insurance for middle-class families who bought it in the individual market could be twice as much as the cost of insurance obtained at work![32] Unfortunately, this inequity will continue for many families under health reform. In addition, a new system of subsidies will create new inequities.

For instance, employees earning $15 an hour can get a federal tax subsidy for family coverage in the exchange that is $13,000 more than the tax subsidy they would receive if they obtain insurance at work. For higher-income workers, the inequity moves in the opposite direction. Someone earning $100,000 can get a tax subsidy for employer-provided coverage that is $10,000 or more. Yet this same employee would get no subsidy if forced to buy health insurance in an exchange.

The subsidies are also arbitrary within the exchange itself. A couple who decides to marry may find they lose more than $1,000 in subsidies as a result.[33] Some middle-age couples will qualify for a larger subsidy than younger families whose income is far lower than theirs.[34] [See, " How Much Will My Health Insurance Cost?" and "Does Marriage Help or Hurt?"]

Access to care may become more difficult for some patients.
Health economists estimate that people with health insurance usually consume twice as much health care as people without it.[35] Thus, within the next few years, millions of newly insured people will probably seek to double their use of health care.[36] Millions of others will be required to obtain insurance that is more generous than what they previously had, and the more generous coverage will also induce them to seek more care.

The result: The demand for medical care is likely to greatly exceed the supply. Though there is disagreement about the size of the coming physician shortage, Medicare's chief actuary and some private sector economists are predicting major problems in access to care, including increased waiting.[37] In Massachusetts, with a similar health reform:

- New patients in Boston wait more than two months, on the average, to see a family doctor.[38]
- More people are going to hospital emergency rooms for nonemergency care than before.[39]

The quality of care may fall rather than rise for average patients. Health reform assumes that people with insurance will be healthier and live longer than people without it. While that seems to be relatively uncontroversial for private insurance, half the newly insured will be enrolling in Medicaid. Do people fare better on Medicaid than they do when they are uninsured? The latest (and best) study of the issue looked at Oregon and found that being in Medicaid made little difference — either for people's health or their life expectancy.[40] [See "What if I have to be in Medicaid?"]

Overall, the evidence shows that private insurance is superior to Medicare and Medicaid.[41] To the degree that the changes push people out of private coverage and into public programs, quality of care may suffer. More worrisome are the across-the-board cuts in Medicare fees called for under the Affordable Care Act. [See "What if I am on Medicare?"]. Indiscriminate changes in Medicare spending seem to have a clear impact on seniors. One study found that a 10 percent increase in Medicare spending leads to a 1.5 percent improvement in odds of survival — and vice versa.[42] A second study found that a 1 percent decrease in Medicare hospital spending led to a 0.4 percent increase in mortality.[43] And a third study estimates that 6,300 additional deaths are likely because of the cuts in Medicare spending over the first 10 years under ObamaCare.[44]

One way the new law addresses the problem of quality is by authorizing pilot programs and demonstration projects. Research funds are to be allocated to discover best practices, and Medicare has new powers to prod doctors and hospitals into changing how they practice medicine. Yet the CBO has found these programs are not working.[45] Many scholars are skeptical that much will come of these efforts.

Meanwhile, serious concerns are arising about the quality of the insurance being sold in the health insurance exchanges. As New York Times reporter Robert Pear has documented, these plans seem to be leaving out the best doctors and the best hospitals and restricting their networks to those providers who will accept low fees.[46] The Mayo Clinic and the Cleveland Clinic are just two examples of centers of excellence that may not be accessible to those who use the exchanges.

Another problem faces those who rely on our safety net institutions. Even if ObamaCare achieves all of its enrollment goals, 30 million people (more than half the total uninsured population) will remain uninsured. Many will turn to the emergency rooms of safety net hospitals when they need medical care. In addition, some studies are finding people who enroll in Medicaid go to hospital emergency rooms more often, not less often. In fact, their ER visits increase by about 40 percent.[47] Yet despite the increased need for resources, the Affordable Care Act is actually reducing federal subsidies for safety net hospitals by billions of dollars.[48]

As noted, the medical community is bracing itself for a major rationing problem: The new health reform law will expand the demand for care, relative to the supply, at almost every hospital and every doctor's office. Designers of the health reform law frequently state their desire to see providers become more efficient. But that is easier said than done. In Britain, Canada and other developed countries, doctors often deal with these problems by reducing the time they spend with each patient.[49]

The Role of Government. By far, the most significant change in health reform will be the new role of government. You, your family and your employer will no longer be able to make many of the decisions you have been making on your own. Instead, the power to make those decisions has been shifted to 159 new federal agencies, exerting unprecedented control over almost one-sixth of the economy. Moreover, the Secretary of Health and Human Services has gained extraordinary discretionary powers. The two acts creating health reform, for example, delegate powers through the phrase "the Secretary shall" 1,075 times.

Federally mandated benefits. Under the new law, all insurance that is not grandfathered must include benefits determined by the federal government. This means you must pay for benefits you may not want or need. Women will have to pay for coverage for prostate cancer tests. Men will have to buy coverage for mammograms. People beyond the child-bearing age will have to buy coverage for maternity care. And teetotalers will have to buy coverage for alcohol and substance abuse.[50]

Less patient power. Employees will not be allowed to make many decisions they are making today. For example, considerable controversy exists over who should get mammograms, Pap smears, prostate cancer tests and other procedures — and at what age and how often.[51] Instead of dictating a one-solution-for-everyone approach, some employers put money in a health savings account for their employees and let them make their own buying decisions. But the new law forbids that flexibility. Instead, a federal advisory panel will determine who is eligible for what test and when, and health plans will be required to cover these services with no deductible or copayment.

Less freedom of medical practice. The federal government will conduct extensive comparative effectiveness research

— evaluating what works, what doesn't work and what's worthwhile. A similar agency in Britain gives local health authorities "cover" to deny patients such care as cancer drugs that are routinely available in the United States and Europe.[52] Critics worry the same could happen here.

Where Will I Get My Health Insurance?

You may get it the same place you get it today — through an employer, Medicare or Medicaid, or through a contractor for one of those programs (such as a private Medicare Advantage plan).

If you buy your own insurance, however, you will have to obtain it through a health insurance exchange in order to be eligible for subsidies. Also, whether you go inside or outside of the exchange, competing insurers will be forced to offer government-mandated packages of benefits.

However, if your income is below 100 percent of the poverty level (currently $11,490 for an individual and $23,550 for a family of four) or if you are eligible for Medicaid (or an affordable employer plan), you will not have access to the exchange.

Will I Be Able to Keep the Insurance I Now Have?

Despite President Obama's promise that "If you like your plan you can keep it," about 6 million people have already been notified by insurance companies that their insurance is being canceled. That number will grow. Currently, about 19 million people have health coverage purchased in the individual market. Most of those plans do not comply with the requirements of the Affordable Care Act. One expert estimates that more than 15 million people will lose their individual insurance by the end of 2014 because of the new law.[53]

The architects of health reform intended this outcome, and the health insurance industry was well aware of the consequences. However, the cancellations are coming as a complete surprise to most individual policyholders.

Technically, anyone who bought insurance prior to the passage of the Affordable Care Act is "grandfathered" and immune from most of the new regulations, as long as the plan stays intact.[54] However, the Obama administration has issued rules and regulations that make it almost impossible for individual insurance policies to remain grandfathered. For example, even small changes in deductibles and copayments or a switch of insurance plans offered by the same carrier means forfeiting grandfathered status. These same regulations have not been applied to large businesses that self-insure for their employees' health benefits.

Administration officials, including President Obama himself, were surprised at the large number of insurance plans that were canceled in the fall of 2013. These cancellations were the direct result of health reform, however, including regulatory decisions that the Obama administration made for the express purpose of forcing people out of the individual market and into the newly created exchanges.[55] [See "What If My Insurance Has Been Canceled?"]

Your Employer May Be Forced to Switch to Another Plan.
In general, if employers make very few changes to their current plan, that plan will be grandfathered. But (even among employers) most plans will not qualify for grandfathered status. A government memorandum predicts that:[56]

- More than half of all employees — and as many as two-thirds — with employer-provided health insurance will have to switch to more expensive, more regulated plans.
- As many as 80 percent of employees in small businesses will be required to switch to other plans.
- Moreover, grandfathering is only a temporary reprieve. The memorandum suggests that eventually all plans will lose their grandfathered status.

A survey of employers by Hewitt suggests that last prediction may be too optimistic: 90 percent of employers expect to lose their grandfathered status. A majority expect to do so before the employer mandate takes effect.[57] [See "Your Employer May Drop Coverage Altogether" below.]

19

Your Employer May Drop Coverage Altogether. By 2016, all but the smallest employers will be required to provide health insurance or pay a fine. But since the fine will be as little as one-seventh of the cost of insuring you and your family, many employers may drop their coverage altogether. In that case, you and other employees will be required to obtain insurance on your own — in the marketplace or in a health insurance exchange.

Private firms that advise employers have indicated that many of their clients would be better off dropping employee coverage.

- The consulting firm Deloitte found one in ten employers planned to drop employee benefits.[58]
- Consulting firm McKinsey & Co. surveyed clients and found that about 30 percent of employers "definitely or probably" would stop offering coverage.[59]

Overall:

- The CBO estimates that 4 million employees will lose their employer plans.[60]
- Medicare's chief actuary estimates that 14 million employees will lose the coverage they now have, and of those, about 2 million will enroll in Medicaid.[61]
- A former CBO director is predicting a much larger employer response, with 35 million employees losing their current coverage.[62]

You Employer May Make You an Offer You Can't Afford to Accept. Employers who are self-insured (and more than half of all employees work for a self-insured employer) have more options. By providing somewhat skimpy insurance—but nonetheless insurance that covers preventive care with no lifetime cap — they can avoid paying a $2,000 fine for each employee. But since this insurance will not satisfy the full requirements of the new law, you may go to the exchange and get subsidized insurance. If you do, your employer will be liable for a $3,000 fine.

Your employer could avoid that fine by offering to "top up" the skimpy insurance to comply with the ACA by requiring you to pay a costly premium equal to 9.5 percent of your annual wage for your coverage, and the full premium for your spouse and children. For a $50,000 wage earner, 9.5 percent is $4,750 — nearly the average cost of covering an employee, according to national surveys. Paying the full cost of covering a family would add more than $10,000 to that total annually. Few workers will be willing to spending half their take-home pay on health insurance — unless they expect some whopping medical bills. But this offer — one almost no worker could afford to accept — would satisfy the employer mandate.

Under the law, to add insult to injury, if you turn down this offer, you will not be entitled to any subsidy if you buy your own insurance in the exchange. [See "What If I Am an Employer?"]

Loss of Medicare Advantage Coverage. About half the enrollees in Medicare Advantage plans (7.5 million people) are likely to lose their coverage and will be forced to return to conventional Medicare.[63] If you are able to keep your Advantage plan, expect higher premiums and fewer benefits because of the cuts in payments to those plans mandated by the new law.

Loss of Post-retirement Coverage. If you are a retiree and your previous employer has supplemental insurance that pays the cost of your drugs, you are unlikely to be able to keep your plan. Under current law, employers receive a direct subsidy plus a tax subsidy if they provide Medicare Part D benefits that the government would otherwise have to pay for. The health reform law removes the tax subsidy, however. As a result, almost all retirees with employer coverage for prescription drugs (5.8 million out of 6.6 million) are expected to eventually lose it, according to the latest Medicare Trustees report.

Loss of Limited Benefit Plans. Millions of Americans had a health insurance plan that features "limited benefits," sometimes called "mini-med" plans. In mini-med plans, medical benefits are capped anywhere from a few thousand dollars to $25,000 or even $50,000 or more annually. Premiums are affordable — a family policy can be as little as $1,000 per year. The Affordable Care Act is designed to ban such plans.

As a temporary measure to delay the loss of health coverage for many workers, the Department of Health and Human Services granted waivers for limited benefit health plans to more than 1,200 companies with more than 4 million employees.[64] The waivers allow these employees to keep their health plans through 2013. Some of the organizations that received waivers were staunch supporters of the health reform bill, including unions such as the Service Employees International Union, the Teamsters, and the United Food and Commercial Workers.

What Will My New Health Insurance Look Like?

All health insurance sold in an exchange must be standardized, covering all of the mandated benefits.[65] The types of plans are labeled Bronze, Silver, Gold and Platinum. The only difference among these plans is the level of cost sharing — less expensive plans have higher deductibles and copayments (see the table) — and smaller networks of doctors and hospitals.

Cost Sharing for Exchange Policies

Plan Type	Percent of Expected Medical Costs Paid by the Plan
Bronze	60%
Silver	70%
Gold	80%
Platinum	90%

Source: Affordable Care Act

CBO estimates originally suggested that the insurance would look a lot like a standard BlueCross plan paying BlueCross fees to providers. This is turning out not to be the case. Insurers have discovered the healthy select policies based on price; the sick tend to want full coverage and access to a full range of providers. Thus, one mechanism to discourage the sick is to feature tight networks. A way to encourage young, healthy individuals to enroll is to offer low prices. As a result of these perverse incentives, we are seeing a race to the bottom on access with private plans in the exchanges looking increasingly like Medicaid.

In California, about 70 percent of physicians either are excluded from networks or declined to join them.[66] This is consistent with the earlier experience of Massachusetts. Subsidized insurance in that state pays provider reimbursement rates that are lower than other private insurance — often between Medicare and Medicaid rates.[67]

Who Can Buy Catastrophic-Only Insurance?

The health reform law allows young people under age 30 access to catastrophic health coverage. These plans must cover three primary care visits along with included preventive services with no deductible. Additional services are covered after the deductible is reached ($6,250 for an individual and $12,500 for a family of four).[68]

By many estimates, the cost of catastrophic coverage is much less. Catastrophic plans have risk pools separate from the more comprehensive "metal plans" and do not have to satisfy 3:1 age band ratings, which require that the premium, say, for a 25-year-old, cannot be less than one-third of the premium for a 60-year-old. Otherwise, premiums for young buyers would be much lower. Unlike the exchange plans, there are no subsidies for catastrophic plans.

In December 2013, the Obama administration announced that people older than 30 who have had their insurance canceled can claim a "hardship exemption," and they too can purchase non-conforming, catastrophic coverage.[69] Insurers fear this will destabilize the market by allowing healthy individuals to escape costly ObamaCare regulations while unhealthy enrollees swell the ranks and boost premiums for more comprehensive health plans.

How Much Will My Health Insurance Cost?

The new law requires most individuals to obtain a health insurance plan beginning this year. The CBO's preliminary analysis estimated the least expensive plan, known as the Bronze plan, would cost $4,500 to $5,000 per year for an individual and $12,000 to $12,500 for a family.[70] The CBO also estimated that, by 2016, typical coverage will average about $5,800 for an individual and $15,000 for a family of four.[71]

The good news: Average premiums in the exchange are 16 percent lower than the CBO's initial projection.[72] The bad news: Deductibles and copayments are higher than what most people are used to, and the network of doctors and hospitals is much narrower. To enroll in a plan with a low deductible and access to most providers, an individual will likely pay a premium much closer to the original CBO estimate.

Your Share of the Cost in the Exchange. Your share of the premium is determined by your income and by the premium charged by a benchmark plan (the second-lowest-priced Silver plan). If you earn 133 percent of the federal poverty level (currently $15,281 for an individual and $31,321 for a family of four), the subsidy will limit the premium you must pay for the benchmark plan to 3 percent of your income. Individuals earning between 100 and 138 percent of the poverty level will also be able to purchase private coverage in the exchange if they are not eligible to enroll in their state's Medicaid program. Their premiums for the benchmark plan will be limited to 2 percent of income. At 400 percent of the federal poverty level (currently $45,960 for an individual and $94,200 for a family of four)., the subsidy will limit the premium you must pay to 9.5 percent of your income. Above that level, you will receive no subsidy, and you will have to pay the full price yourself. [See the tables below.]

The benchmark plan is used to determine the federal subsidy you are entitled to. However, you are free to choose other, more expensive Silver plans or Gold and Platinum plans. If you do choose a more expensive plan, you must pay the full cost of the extra expense.

Net Cost of Health Insurance after Subsidies

Income Level	Permium as a Percent of Income*
Up to 133% FPL	2% of Income
133% - 150% FPL	3-4% of Income
150% - 200% FPL	4-6.3% of Income
200% - 250% FPL	6.3-8.05% of Income
250% - 300% FPL	8.05-9.5% of Income
300% - 400% FPL	9.5% of Income
*For the benchmark plan only	

Source: Department of Health and Human Services

2013 Federal Poverty Guidelines

Household Size	100%	133%	400%
1	$11,490	$15,282	$45,960
2	$15,510	$20,628	$62,040
3	$19,530	$25,975	$78,120
4	$23,550	$31,322	$94,200
5	$27,570	$36,668	$110,280
6	$31,590	$42,015	$126,360
7	$35,610	$47,361	$142,440
8	$39,360	$52,708	$158,520
For each additional person, add	$4,020	$5,347	$16,080

Source: Department of Health and Human Services

How Is Income Determined? Your subsidy in the exchange will be based on your modified adjusted gross income (MAGI) — your adjusted gross income with certain deductions added back, including: deductions for student-loan payments, IRA-contributions and spending on higher-education. The state and federal health exchanges were supposed to be able to verify income by linking to the IRS. However, since the interface is not working, people are being asked to report their income more or less on the honor system — not their "MAGI," just their "income." This almost guarantees that all the income numbers will be wrong, however. To make matters worse, everyone has an incentive to underreport their income in order to get higher subsidies.

What Happens if the Subsidy You Receive Is the Wrong Amount? If it turns out that your 2014 subsidy was too high, given your actual income that year, the IRS will be able to reclaim part of the unwarranted portion by collecting additional taxes from you the following year. If it turns out that your subsidy was too low, you can file for a refund for the amount of the underpayment.

Strangely, these outcomes are not symmetrical. The IRS can reclaim only limited amounts from most people (up to $300 in overpayments for an individual and $600 for families earning less than 200 percent of poverty; $2,500 for families earning between 300 and 400 percent of poverty; unlimited for those earning more than 400 percent).[73] However, there is no limit on the underpayments you can reclaim from the IRS.

How Subsidies Affect Your Marginal Tax Rate. As your income rises, the subsidy falls, and the premium you must pay rises. This rising premium is like a tax, and the marginal rate will be very high. When the effects of the subsidy withdrawals are added to income and payroll taxes, most people will lose more than 50 cents for each $1 they earn.[74]

A New Hampshire couple, Doug and Ginger Chapman, found that earnings just above the subsidy limit can be costly. Because their income was just above the threshold, they did not qualify for subsidies. The lowest cost for health coverage they found was about $12,000 per year. Had they earned a few thousand less, they would have qualified for a subsidy that would have cut their annual insurance bill nearly in half.[75] Had they earned less than 400 percent of poverty ($94,200 for a family of four), their premiums would have been limited to 9.5 percent of income. In this example, $6,000 in income boosts premium costs by nearly $6,000 — effectively imposing a marginal tax rate of nearly 100 percent!

Are You Entitled to a Subsidy if the Exchange Is Run by the Federal Government? Although the health care law establishes generous subsidies for health coverage purchased in state-based health insurance exchanges, it makes no provision for subsidies in the 35 health insurance exchanges run by the federal government. The IRS has indicated that it will interpret the law so that subsidies will be available to applicants in both federally run and state-based exchanges. However, some policy analysts and members of Congress question whether that interpretation is legal, and the issue is currently being litigated in the courts.[76]

Who Runs the Exchanges In Your State?

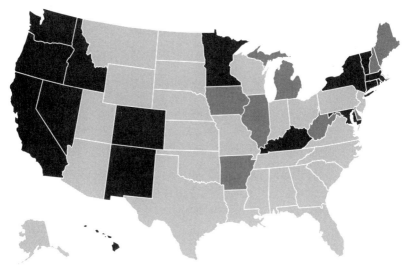

- Federally-run exchange
- Federally-run exchange in partnership with a state
- State-run exchange

Source: Kaiser Family Foundation

Your Share of the Premium at Work. If your wage income from your employer is less than 400 percent of poverty, your share of the premium will be limited to no more than 9.5 percent of your wage income. There is a big difference between the limits in the exchange and the limits at work, however. In the exchange, your share of the premium (for the benchmark plan) will be kept low by a refundable tax credit — a gift from the government that will pay the remaining premium expenses. For most employer coverage, no new subsidies will apply. If your employer is required to reduce the amount of the premium you pay at work, he will likely make up the extra cost by reducing other compensation (cash wages and other benefits). In the exchange, the government pays to keep your premium low; but at work, it's likely that you will pay.

Smoking and Wellness Programs. Health plans and employers spend about $6 billion annually on health and wellness programs. Hundreds of vendors compete for this business, and the Affordable Care Act is likely to boost that number. Under the new rules, health plans may refund up to 30 percent of the total cost of coverage for participation in wellness programs. The Department of Health and Human Services has the authority to authorize even higher rewards — up to 50 percent discounts for well-designed programs.

For example, say an employee health plan costs $6,000, to which an employee contributes $1,500. If the employee participates in a wellness program, the employer plan could refund $1,800 to the employee — 30 percent of the $6,000 premium cost.[77]

If you smoke, don't be surprised if your health plan penalizes you with a surcharge of up to 50 percent in higher premiums. Again, this calculation is based on the total cost of a health plan, not just your contribution. Using the previous example, a worker who smokes could be penalized $3,000 in higher premiums on a plan that costs $6,000 — tripling the employee's contribution!

However, an employer can also reward you with discounts of 20 to 50 percent of premiums for participating in smoking cessation programs. This means a plan could charge smokers extra but give back some or all of the penalty to those participating in a smoking cessation program. Not all states allow smoking surcharges, and many insurers don't want to run the risk of driving away business by charging higher premiums to smokers.

Wellness programs must be reasonably designed not to discriminate against enrollees by health status. For example, a program could reward enrollees for participating in an activity, such as walking, running or exercising, but accommodations must be made for people who cannot participate due to a health condition.[78] An employer can offer a reward for participating in a weight-loss program, for instance, but cannot make the reward contingent solely upon a participant actually losing weight. Rather, employers are required to allow enrollees to receive the reward just for participating, providing multiple ways to qualify for the reward.

Unequal Subsidies. As the table below shows, government provides very different subsidies, depending on your income and where you acquire health insurance. In general, the new system is more generous to lower-income families if they obtain insurance in the exchange and is more generous to higher-income families if they obtain insurance at work. Some of these differences are strange:

- A family earning $30,000 per year will get a $19,400 subsidy (covering most of the premium for the benchmark plan plus most out-of-pocket expenses) if purchasing coverage in the exchange, but only $2,811 for coverage through an employer.

- A family earning $60,000 per year will get $12,400 if purchasing coverage in the exchange, more than four times the subsidy available to a family with half as much income getting insurance at work.

- A family earning $90,100 per year will get $3,900 if purchasing coverage in the exchange, nearly 40 percent more than the subsidy available to a family earning one-third as much and getting insurance at work.

Health Reform Tax Subsidies in 2016

Income (AGI)	Subsidy In the Exchange	Subsidy at Work
$30,000	$19,400	$2,811
42,000	17,400	3,921
54,000	14,300	4,497
66,000	10,500	4,796
78,000	6,700	4,661
90,100	3,900	4,545
102,100	0	4,545

Sources: National Center for Policy Analysis/Congressional Budget Office/Joint Committee on Taxation

Is There a Risk of Death Spiral? Insurance companies fear that too many enrollees will have high health care costs, and too few will be basically healthy. If that happens, the insurers will have to raise their premiums. But those circumstances will make insurance even less attractive to people with moderate medical expenses. If more of them drop out, premiums must be raised even more. Eventually, premiums could spiral up so high that no one can afford them. At that point the insurance companies go bankrupt or leave the market.

Six factors cause concern.

First, signing up on the Internet has proved very difficult. The original designers expected signup would take seven minutes. In fact, the average signup time is closer to 45 minutes, and some people have been unable to enroll after many, many hours of trying.[79] Thus, insurers worry that this lengthy and arduous process has already discouraged all but the most desperate customers—the ones expecting to need the most medical care.

Second, because the state high-risk pools are slated to end, states will dump their enrollees into the new exchanges. And about 107,000 people who have been in the federal high-risk pool for people with pre-existing conditions will join them.

Third, many cash-strapped cities, counties and public entities are planning to reduce their unfunded obligations by ending their retiree health plans and sending the retirees to the exchanges. For instance, the city of Detroit — with more than 19,000 retirees — is currently in bankruptcy. Chicago also is reportedly looking into ways to send some of its nearly 12,000 retirees — many of whom are too young to be eligible for Medicare — into the exchange.

Fourth, employers are also looking for ways to lower the medical bills it picks up for retired employees. IBM announced it would end employee health benefits for its 110,000 retirees by 2014.[80] Indeed, a survey by employee benefits consulting firm Towers Watson found that nearly half of mid-size and large employers may discontinue health care benefits for pre-and post-65 retirees.[81] Since expected health costs rise with age, these enrollees will have above-average costs.

Fifth, millions of people have been "locked in" to their jobs — working only to get employer-provided health insurance because a pre-existing condition prevents them from buying affordable health insurance in the individual market.[82] The new law frees these high-cost individuals to leave their empoyer and buy coverage in the exchanges.

Sixth, there is a worry that employers will game the new system. If they have basically healthy employees, they can self-insure (keep their employees in a pool of their own) and avoid the costs of more widespread community rating. However, if their workforce becomes significantly less healthy, they can end their insurance, pay a fine and send the employees to get (possibly subsidized) insurance in the exchange. This kind of gaming will increase costs within the exchange. [See "What If I Am An Employer?"]

Increases in Costs Over Time. Even if a death spiral is avoided, a long-term problem is built into the health reform law. People will be forced to buy insurance, the cost of which is going to grow faster than their income. In fact, if we stay on the path we have traveled for the past 40 years, health care costs (and, therefore, premiums) will rise at twice the rate of growth of our incomes.

In the past, individuals and their employers have done a number of things to try to control their health insurance costs. These include higher deductibles, health savings accounts (which allow you to manage your own small-dollar expenses), more limited benefits or even a shift to catastrophic-only insurance. However, many of these responses will be curtailed under the reform. Out-of-pocket spending (on covered items) is limited, for example, and preventive services must be available with no deductible or copayment.

Also, after 2018, the subsidies in the exchanges will grow no faster than the rate of growth of the economy from year to year. But if we return to historical trends, the cost of health insurance will grow twice as fast.

What If I Am in a Union?

Labor unions were early supporters of ObamaCare. However, union officials are beginning to regret that decision.[83]   About 21 million workers belong to multiemployer unions. These workers typically work for many small employers rather than a single employer, and the unions bargain industrywide with the employers over wages and benefits. They include carpenters, plumbers, roofers, performing artists, metal workers and even members of the Teamsters union. The agreements are called Taft-Hartley plans, and they include reasonably good health insurance.

Here's the problem. These union members are competing against nonunion workers, who also work for small employers but who usually don't receive health insurance as part of their work arrangement. The Affordable Care Act did nothing for the union workers. But it's a godsend for their nonunion competitors, who can now go into the exchanges and get subsidized insurance. Moreover, since the union workers pay taxes (just like everybody else), they are helping to subsidize the insurance of the nonunion competitors.

It gets worse.

Union plans (along with other self-insured plans) pay a small tax that subsidizes health plans sold in the exchange. This annual fee (the so-called "belly button tax," but more technically a "reinsurance fee") is a $63 tax imposed on each person covered by the union health plan. Former Bush administration official Doug Badger says another way to look at the belly button tax is to see it as a $10 billion tax on people who will not get coverage through the exchange paid to those who do.[84]

The Obama administration recently granted some union plans an exemption from the $63 belly button tax.[85] However, the Obama administration angered the union chiefs when it decided unions' special Taft-Hartley plans are ineligible for exchange subsidies.[86]

How Do Health Insurance Exchanges Work?

A health insurance exchange is an artificial market where insurance plans compete for customers, usually during an annual enrollment period called an open season. Federal employees, for example, get their health insurance this way. The federal government pays about 75 percent of the cost, and the employees pay the other 25 percent, typically choosing from a dozen or so plans. Many employees of state and local governments, including many public colleges and universities, also participate in health insurance exchanges. In addition, a few states (e.g., Massachusetts and Utah) have established exchanges for broad-based populations. The Massachusetts plan is allegedly the model on which the new federal health reform law is based.

Unlike the system for federal employees, however, insurers in the new ObamaCare state-based exchanges must offer the same basic package of benefits, although they may differ in how those benefits are provided. For example, some plans may be health maintenance organizations (HMOs), while others have provider networks. Plans may also differ with respect to deductibles and copayments.

Attractive Features of Exchanges. Competition and choice must rank high on the list of favorable features. The exchanges are designed to function as one-stop shops where consumers can compare competing health plans. The state and federal websites are designed to steer applicants to public plans that they may qualify for and to assess financial need and subsidies available. Plans must charge everyone of the same age the same premium, regardless of health status. Moreover, plans have standardized benefit levels so shoppers have a better idea of the benefits they are comparing. In theory, exchange plans should contain fewer surprises, so that enrollees aren't surprised to learn a service isn't covered.

Unattractive Features of Exchanges. Offsetting these benefits are some negative features:

Opportunities for people to game the system. Federal and state employee exchanges cater to self-contained groups. Employees rarely go outside of the exchange (because they can't use their employer subsidy on the outside), and outsiders (nonemployees) can't get in. In a system-wide exchange (like Massachusetts), however, people have perverse incentives to game the system. They can remain uninsured while they are healthy (paying a small fine, perhaps), then enroll in a health plan after they get sick, get their health care, get their medical bills paid, and drop their coverage once they get well.

In Massachusetts, these so-called "jumpers" and "dumpers" buy into a plan when they have a health problem, then stop paying premiums and dump the plan when the need is gone.

Of course, if everyone does this, only sick people will be paying premiums, and that premium will be very high. Further, as the premiums rise, the least sick people (for whom insurance is only marginally valuable) drop out, leaving the pool sicker and more expensive than it was before. Eventually this "death spiral" will bankrupt all the insurers, unless something is done to prevent it. [See "How Much Will My Health Insurance Cost?"]

In the ACA exchanges, mechanisms have been created to redistribute money from profitable insurers to unprofitable ones. In addition, money has been set aside to subsidize insurance industry profits for the first three years. Even with the subsidies, however, private insurers cannot survive a true death spiral.

Opportunities for insurance companies to game the system. Health plans make profits on healthy enrollees and lose money on sick ones. Since buyers in the exchange pay community-rated premiums that cannot vary with the enrollees' expected medical costs, insurers have perverse incentives to find ways to attract the healthy and avoid the sick.

To a small degree, the effects of these incentives can be seen in the federal employees' health plan.[87] However, because of intense federal pressure to keep premiums low along with efforts to promote vigorous competition, the effects of these incentives are becoming much more pronounced in the ObamaCare exchanges. As noted, insurers expect healthy applicants to care far more about price than about access to a broad network of doctors and hospitals. By contrast, people with chronic conditions and costly health problems are likely to be willing to pay more for comprehensive health plans with low cost sharing and access to broad networks. Thus, many of the health plans in the exchanges feature high-deductibles and narrow networks, while in many places, Platinum health plans are not available at all.

The changing nature of insurance. Remember the TV ads that end with the statement, "You're in good hands with Allstate"? These ads ask you to focus on how the insurer will treat you if something goes wrong. They promise you that you will get really good treatment if you are ever unlucky enough to need the insurer to pay claims. Federal employees almost never see health insurance ads like this. During the open season, for example, insurance company advertisements tend to picture young, healthy families with children. They never mention what happens if you are unlucky enough to have heart disease, cancer or AIDS. That's because health insurers don't want enrollees who pay average premiums but have expensive-to-treat problems. Since there are no pre-existing illness limitations in an exchange, the healthy employees may assume that if they ever get sick, they can always switch to a plan that is good at treating their particular illness. Unfortunately, they may find out too late that plans skilled in treating expensive problems have been driven from the market.

The effects of low reimbursement rates. In Massachusetts, subsidized health plans are paying low provider fees, usually similar to Medicaid and Medicare rates. Nationwide, Medicare pays doctors only about 80 percent of what a private insurer would pay for the same service; Medicaid pays about 60 percent. Since the rates paid by exchange plans are well below the market rates, doctors are likely to see private-paying patients first and then Medicare patients — pushing patients with exchange plans to the rear of the waiting lines.

What If the Exchange in My State Isn't Ready?

Why Weren't the Exchanges Ready on Time? On October 1, 2013, millions of Americans were supposed to be able to go online and acquire health insurance on electronic exchanges in the states where they live. But the exchanges weren't ready. The Department of Health and Human Services has already thrown in the towel on small-business exchanges, which were supposed to allow employees to choose among competing health plans. For most employees, the opportunity to make those choices has been put off for at least a year, leaving them with only their employer's plans as options. Individuals acquiring insurance on their own have faced great difficulties — as we have seen.

More than one commentator has remarked on the puzzling way the Obama presidency has dealt with online technology. When it came to elections, the Obama campaign's use of the Internet was state of the art — doing what had never been done before. Yet when it came to the health insurance exchanges, the administration has been using 10-year-old technology — producing a website with defects that are baffling to a whole generation of website designers.

The short explanation seems to be that President Obama privatized his election campaigns, while he nationalized health reform. The Internet aspect of his election campaign was managed by experts from Google and other entrepreneurial ventures, who were able to devise strategies unencumbered by bureaucrats in Washington, D.C. In designing the health insurance exchanges, by contrast, almost everything has been managed top down from Washington, D.C. (with 55 contractors separately reporting to the agency in charge).[88]

Prior to the Affordable Care Act, the only states that had functioning exchanges were Massachusetts and Utah. Both developed their exchanges independently of the Affordable Care Act, and their exchanges are not able to do everything the federal government requires. Fifteen states and the District of Columbia operate their own exchanges with varying degrees of success. The remaining states have either completely ceded responsibility to the federal government or have entered a partnership that gives the federal government responsibility.[89]

Three problems are evident.

First, too little money was budgeted for creating the exchanges. The CBO originally estimated that setting up the exchanges would cost $5 to $10 billion. California alone has spent more than $900 million. Yet the health reform law allocated only $1 billion for the entire country.

A second problem is complexity. The Obama administration tried to create something the federal government has never done: a computer system that connects the Department of Health and Human Services, the Internal Revenue Service, the Social Security Administration, Homeland Security and perhaps other departments. This is a herculean task.

A third and much bigger problem is competency. The federal government is probably the worst entity possible to design such an exchange. The federal government has tried to reinvent systems the private sector has already, quite competently, created. But true to form, in designing ObamaCare, government completely ignored private exchanges that have been up and running, in some cases for more than a decade.[90]

For example, over many years, the Department of Defense and the Department of Veterans Affairs spent $1.3 billion trying to develop a shared electronic medical records system.[91] After many technological challenges and innumerable delays, the agencies ultimately abandoned the project.[92]

What If I have trouble signing up? You have several options. Even before the exchanges became available, some states (Texas is a notable example) allowed residents who renewed coverage

37

before the end of 2013 to retain it through 2014. In many cases, this allowed individuals to avoid the higher-cost exchange plans for one more year. As the state and federal exchanges experienced problems, both the president and the Secretary of Health and Human Services announced in mid-November 2013 that states had the discretion to allow individuals to retain their current coverage for one more year. Not all state insurance commissioners allow this. And where they do allow it, the insurance companies may decline.

To learn if you can continue your previous coverage, begin by contacting your insurance agent or the company that provided your health plan in 2013.

Another resource is eHealth.com, an independent website that sells health coverage offered by numerous insurers, including Aetna, BlueCross and Cigna. You can avoid HealthCare.gov (and your state exchange) and contact an insurer directly — although these plans will not qualify for subsidies. Also, check with officials in your state to see if a nonprofit organization in your area employs individuals (called "navigators") to assist people in signing up. People can call the federal hot line (1-800-318-2596) if they cannot get through on the website.

What If My Insurance Has Been Canceled?

Nearly 6 million people had their health insurance canceled in 2013, and the number is likely to exceed 15 million by the end of 2014. The cancellations occurred because these plans did not conform to ObamaCare mandated benefits. In other cases, state law is the culprit. For example, as a contractual condition of selling health plans in the California exchange, CoveredCalifornia, insurers were required to cancel existing policies and force those already covered into the exchange.

As a result, many people had no health insurance for a period of time, because they had difficulty obtaining insurance that became effective January 1.

Why would regulations whose ostensible goal is universal

health coverage do things to cause millions of people to lose their insurance?[93]   Both in Washington and at the state level, regulators sympathetic to ObamaCare believed that forcing insurers to drop existing policies and bringing all people currently insured into the exchange would make health plans sold in the exchange financially secure. Their concern was that healthy people with existing coverage in 2013, would retain their old plan if it was cheaper than the new exchange plans. If this healthier group were allowed to continue with lower-cost plans, the only people in the exchange would be high-cost enrollees. This could destabilize the exchange plans and send them into an adverse-selection death spiral. Thus, many state officials wanted to shut down the old plans — even before the new exchanges were up and running.

On November 14, 2013, the Department of Health and Human Services sent a letter to state insurance commissioners giving them the discretion to allow individuals to keep their prior coverage for one more year.[94] And nearly three-fourths of states agreed to allow insurers to reinstate canceled health plans. However, it appears that most insurers are not taking them up on the offer. Indeed, the practice has been specifically a barred in a handful of states, including Washington, Indiana and the District of Columbia.[95]

Consumers gained an 11th-hour reprieve that also allows them to purchase some non-conforming health plans, such as low-cost, catastrophic plans.[96] The administration has also waved the mandate for individuals affected for one more year. [See "What If the Exchange in My State Isn't Ready" and "Who Can Buy Catastrophic Insurance?"]

What If I Am a Member of a Covered Worker's Family?

Employers must offer coverage to workers and their families. Yet, there are no penalties if family coverage is unaffordable. For coverage available at work, the income-based premium limits are based on each worker's wages and the cost of single-only coverage.

An employer plan is still considered affordable in the exchange, even if a one-income family has to pay more than 9.5 percent of family income for a family plan.[97] Once an employer plan meets the definition of affordable and is offered to employees and their families, no member of the family qualifies for subsidized coverage in the exchange — even if they turn the employer offer down.

Calculating Affordable Coverage

	Employee's Premium	Cost of Insurance
Employee's Coverage	$4,720*	$5,000
Remaining family coverage	$10,000	$10,000
	$14,720	$15,000
***9.5% of $50,000**		

Source: Author's calculations

The table shows an example of a $50,000-a-year employee who is asked to pay 9.5 percent of his or her annual gross wage for individual coverage and the full cost of coverage for a spouse and children. Under the law, this is deemed "affordable," even though the employee's share of the total premium is almost 30 percent of his gross wage and almost 40 percent of take home pay. [See "What If I Am An Employer?"]

If the family turns down this offer, they will not be entitled to subsidized health insurance in the exchange.

Are We Being Forced to Buy the Wrong Kind of Insurance?

Many low-income workers have "mini-med" health insurance plans, paid for by their employers. A typical plan limits the health insurance benefit to $2,000. But some companies give employees the option to pay a higher premium and get $3,000 or $4,000 of coverage. Some plans have much higher benefits; for example, TennCare mini-med plans had a $25,000 annual benefit cap.

Mini-med plans typically have no deductible. They usually charge a modest copayment for physician visits and drugs. But if a plan enrollee goes into a hospital, the co-insurance rate is 30 percent, and the benefits will probably be exhausted 30 minutes after admission.

The ACA has abolished these plans, and if the employees end up in one of the new exchanges, their subsidized insurance will look very different. Premiums could double. Then they will face, say, a $1,500 deductible for individual coverage. Surprisingly, if such an employee goes into a hospital, he or she faces a 20 percent copayment up to the limits on total out-of-pocket spending (currently no more than $6,350 for an individual and $12,700 for a family.

Now, which of these plans is better? Low- and moderate-income households would find the mini-med plan more attractive, because people living paycheck to paycheck have trouble maintaining a reserve for unexpected medical expenses. So as an alternative to personal savings and higher wages, they are willing to trade less take-home pay for a modest amount of health insurance.

How Will the Government Enforce the Requirement to Buy Insurance?

The IRS will serve as the enforcer of health reform. How?

On your annual tax return, you will be required to show proof that you and other members of your family have the minimum insurance the government requires almost everyone to buy. Failure to provide such proof will subject you to tax penalties. Further, providing false information (claiming you have insurance when you don't) will subject you to the same penalties that would apply to other types of false IRS reporting.

Some analysts estimate the IRS will need to hire 16,000 additional agents to fully enforce the requirement that everyone obtain individual health insurance, though the agency has not confirmed this estimate.[98] The president's budget includes a request for 1,954 positions to ensure compliance and verify eligibility.[99]

Many experts believe the mandate will be widely ignored. Failing to purchase health insurance is not considered a crime, nor can you be put in jail. The IRS can withhold your tax refund if you do not have health insurance, but it cannot garnish your wages or place a lien on your property.[100]

What If I Am Uninsured?

In 2014, if you fail to show proof that you have insurance on your income tax return, you will pay a fine of $95 ($285 per family) or 1 percent of income, whichever is greater. For example, the maximum a family earning $50,000 would pay for not having health coverage is $500. Fines will rise to $695 ($2,085 per family) or 2.5 percent of your adjusted gross income, whichever is greater, by 2016.

Among those who are either excluded from the mandate or exempt from the fine are the Amish, Mennonites, prisoners, illegal immigrants and members of American Indian tribes. The mandate also doesn't apply to you if:[101]

- Your income is so low you are not required to file a tax return.
- Your income is below 100 percent of poverty, but you don't have access to Medicaid [See "What If I Have to Be in Medicaid?"]
- You are a family member of a worker who is offered affordable individual coverage by an employer, but you face family premiums in excess of 8 percent of family income.

You can get an exemption if you become homeless; were evicted in the past six months or face eviction or foreclosure; received a shut-off notice from a utility company; recently experienced domestic violence; recently experienced the death of a close family member; recently experienced a fire, flood or other natural or human-caused disaster that resulted in substantial damage to your property; filed for bankruptcy within the last six months; incurred unreimbursed medical expenses in the last 24 months that resulted in substantial debt; or experienced unexpected increases in essential expenses due to caring for an ill, disabled or aging family member.[102]

Can I Keep My Doctor?

Maybe not. You may end up in a plan that restricts your choice of doctors. Or your doctor may end up in a plan that restricts his or her choice of patients. Also, the demand for doctor services will greatly exceed supply — creating new rationing problems.

Plans Sold in the Health Insurance Exchanges. Many health plans sold in the exchanges appear to offer very narrow networks with limited choice of doctors.[103] For example, 70 percent of California physicians are not in CoveredCalifornia exchange plan networks.[104] Moreover, instead of choosing doctors based on the quality of care they deliver, the exchange networks appear to include doctors who are willing to accept the low fees insurers are offering to pay. In some cases, these fees are lower than what Medicare pays.

Employer Plans. Employers also seem to be experimenting with narrow networks. One increasingly popular technique is called "reference pricing." For example, WellPoint selected 46 California hospitals that frequently performed hip and knee replacements for $30,000 or less. Then the insurers told California workers, retired public employees and their families that if they went outside this network, they would have to pay any cost above $30,000.[105]

What If There Aren't Enough Doctors? If government estimates are correct, about 25 million uninsured people will eventually acquire health insurance.[106] If economic studies are correct, the newly insured will try to double their consumption of health care.[107]

In addition to the newly insured, many people will be required to buy health plans with more generous coverage than they have today. All told, as many as 100 million people may acquire health insurance benefits they do not have today.[108] Moreover, most of the other 200 million Americans will be entitled to preventive services without copayments and deductibles they used to face. These people will still expect annual physicals, mammograms, Pap smears, prostate cancer (PSA) tests, colonoscopies and other services. Yet with no increase in supply, there is no realistic way for doctors to meet this demand. [See, "What About Preventive Care?"]

A government website claims funds set aside in the Affordable Care Act will train 16,000 new providers by 2015.[109] But this number appears to count students who are already in medical school—who will simply replace doctors who were expected to retire — and in any event Congress has never appropriated the funds. In fact, all funds for training new providers were eliminated before the health reform law was passed (an effort on the part of Congress to keep spending down). Instead, Health and Human Services Secretary Kathleen Sebelius plans to use $250 million targeted for "prevention and public health" to train 500 physicians, 600 physician assistants and 600 nurse practitioners.[110] Also, she plans to use an additional $500 million of stimulus money available under the American Recovery and Investment Act. Even so, the additional supply will still fall far short of the need.

The Association of American Medical Colleges predicts a shortfall of 21,000 primary care physicians by 2015, and the Health Resources and Services Administration estimates a shortage of between 55,000 and 150,000 physicians by 2020 — and those estimates came before health care reform passed![111] Texas alone is predicting a shortage of 18,000 nurses by 2015.[112]

How Will Doctors Decide Which Patients to Treat? When demand for care expands faster than the supply of doctors, practicing physicians must decide which patients they see first. You will be at a disadvantage if you are in a health plan that pays below-market rates. Nationwide:[113]

- Medicare pays doctors about 19 percent less than private plans.
- Medicaid pays about 28 percent less than Medicare.
- Subsidized plans in the Massachusetts health insurance exchange (the model for the new federal law) pay doctors rates that vary between Medicare and Medicaid rates, and this practice may be repeated in other state exchanges.

What About Hospital Emergency Rooms? Because of the access-to-care problems, the National Center for Policy Analysis and other researchers predict a substantial increase in the number of patients who seek care in hospital emergency rooms.[114]

In general, emergency room use by the uninsured and the privately insured is about the same. Medicaid enrollees, on the other hand, make more than twice as many visits, and about half of all newly insured people will be enrolled in Medicaid.[115] Consequently, the NCPA projects that enrolling 16 million to 18 million new people in Medicaid will generate *between 848,000 and 901,000 additional emergency room visits every year.*

Will My Relationship with My Doctor Change?

It may.

Unanswered Questions. Here are just a few of the questions patients are asking about health reform:

- Will I be able to choose the doctor who treats me, or will I have to accept whatever doctor is available — the way it works in a hospital emergency room?
- Will I be required to stay in a network of doctors, or will I be free to see doctors outside the network?
- Will there be a limit on the number of times I can see a doctor?
- Will doctors be pressured to limit the time they spend with me?
- Will doctors be free to prescribe the drugs I need, the tests I require and the procedures that are indicated?
- Will doctors be free to exercise their best judgment in treating me? Or will doctors be forced to conform to guidelines written by people who may be more concerned with controlling costs than curing disease, treating illness and saving lives?

At this point, the answers largely depend on what health plan you select, what health plan your employer offers you, or how your (private) Medicaid contractor operates. In the future, the answers may also depend on what actions the federal government takes.

One thing is certain. Increasingly, doctors are abandoning their private practices and becoming employees of hospitals. They cite problemswithgruelingworkschedules,inadequatereimbursements and lack of autonomy. The Medical Group Management Association found a 75 percent increase in doctors working for hospitals since 2000; indeed, nearly half of all doctors no longer work for themselves. Doctors who work for hospitals tend to reduce their workload and cut back on patient care — which exacerbates the shortage problem.[116] Another problem is that patients are sometimes discovering — after receiving a large medical bill — that their physician sold his or her practice to a hospital, which usually charges more for the same service. The fees private insurers pay hospitals are anywhere from 5 to 40 percent higher. A patient who has not yet met his or her deductible might face sticker shock.[117]

Vision of the Supporters of Reform. Some of the supporters of the Affordable Care Act have been very explicit. Harvard Medical School professor Atul Gawande, for example, thinks that medicine should be more like engineering — with all doctors following the same script, rather than exercising their individual judgment:[118]

> This can no longer be a profession of craftsmen individually brewing plans for whatever patient comes through the door. We have to be more like engineers building a mechanism whose parts actually fit together, whose workings are ever more finely tuned and tweaked forever better performance in providing aid and comfort to human beings.

Karen Davis, president of the nonprofit Commonwealth Fund, envisions a complete reorganization of the practice of medicine:[119]

> The legislation also includes physician payment reforms that encourage physicians, hospitals, and other providers to join together to form accountable care organizations [ACOs] to gain efficiencies and improve quality of care. Those that meet quality-of-care targets and reduce costs relative to a spending benchmark can share in the savings they generate for Medicare.

Worries of the Critics of Reform. Critics worry that, in actual practice, reform efforts will fall very short of the goals; that practice guidelines will resemble cookbook recipes, rather than representing the best that medicine has to offer. And while these recipes may work for most patients, doctors will not feel free to make exceptions for those who don't fit the norm. Rather than resemble a finely honed machine, the health care system will come to resemble the U.S. Postal Service — even more than it already does.

For example, the ACA encourages the creation of Accountable Care Organizations (ACOs) to deliver care. ACOs have been described as "HMOs on steroids." On paper, it sounds as though doctors working for ACOs will be rewarded for providing higher-quality services. In practice, doctors may be rewarded for underproviding care, just as traditional HMOs were accused of doing.

Moreover, the entire business model of the ACO requires that patients see only the doctors the ACO employs. If you are getting care from an ACO, therefore, your insurance may not pay for you to see outside doctors. Also, part of the ACO vision is that all doctors and nurses will practice medicine in the same way. This means that when you visit a clinic you will not necessarily see the same doctor you saw on your last visit. ACOs will probably be given a lot of freedom to limit the terms and circumstances under which you can see doctors.

Where Private Insurance Is Headed. Even if you are not enrolled in a traditional HMO or an ACO, you can expect a return to some of the heavy-handed health insurance industry practices that were so unpopular in the 1990s and gave rise to the "patient bill of rights" proposals.[120] The reason? The new health care reform takes away just about every other tool insurers have to control costs. In response to the new law, for example, health insurers are already trying to keep premiums down by offering policies that cover, say, only half the doctors in the area where you live.[121] In some of these plans, you get no reimbursement whatsoever if you see a doctor outside the insurer's network.

Levers of Government Power: Medicare. Will the federal government be able to tell doctors how to practice medicine? The designers of health reform quite deliberately set out to change what most doctors do. Reform, for example, will push doctors in Medicare to use electronic medical records, join group practices and ultimately join ACOs. Doctors who do these things will be paid more. Doctors who don't will be paid less. In addition:

- The Federal Coordinating Council for Comparative Effectiveness Research will study alternative ways to treat various conditions, and Medicare itself could refuse to pay doctors and hospitals that do not follow the guidelines.

- There will almost certainly be national guidelines governing who should get diagnostic tests, under what conditions and how often. Medicare doctors are likely to have much less discretion about such diagnostic tests as mammograms, Pap smears, PSA tests, colonoscopies and so on.
- Doctors are also likely to have much less freedom to order CT scans, MRI scans, PET scans, sonograms and other tests.

Levers of Government Power: The Private Sector. The government will have less control over the way doctors practice medicine for privately insured patients. However, health plans in the exchange will face competitive pressures to limit what they spend on people with expensive health problems. Undoubtedly, federal guidelines for Medicare will lead these plans to adopt the same payment strategies for physicians seeing the privately insured. Ultimately, whatever happens under Medicare is likely to spread to the entire private sector.

What Other Countries Have Done. President Obama has said many times that the overriding problem in health care is cost. Health care spending is rising at twice the rate of growth of incomes. If this trend continues, the cost of health care will eventually crowd out every other form of consumption. In this respect, the experience of the United States is not worse than that of other countries. In fact, the real rate of growth of per capita health care spending is just below the average for all developed countries.[122] What makes our country different is that our government has been less involved in cost control efforts.

How have other countries tried to control health care spending? In general, they substitute inexpensive services for expensive ones. Citizens of Britain and Canada, for example, see physicians more often than we do. But as the graph below (page 51) shows, doctors in other countries spend less time with patients on each visit. Also, patients in Britain and Canada have less access to diagnostic tests, even though on paper they are supposed to get all the health care they need for free. Surprisingly, uninsured Americans appear to get as much or more preventive care than insured Canadians. [See the graphs on pages 51-53.]

What About Preventive Care?

The new health care law promises Medicare enrollees annual wellness exams, mammograms, prostate cancer screenings and other preventive services — without any copayment or deductible. The rest of the population will also have access to a lengthy list of preventive services. Unfortunately, the law that mandated these benefits contained no provision that assures doctors will be able to supply them.

What Services Will I Be Entitled To? Since September 23, 2010, all health plans (that were not grandfathered) have been required to cover the preventive services recommended by the U.S. Preventive Services Task Force without cost-sharing. Depending on your age and sex, the following preventive services should be covered by your health insurance:[123]

- Blood pressure, diabetes and cholesterol screening
- Cancer screenings
- Counseling on weight loss, healthy eating, smoking cessation, alcohol use and depression
- Vaccines for measles, polio, meningitis and the human papillomavirus (HPV)
- Shots for flu and pneumonia prevention
- Screening, vaccines and counseling for healthy pregnancies
- Well-baby and well-child visits up to the age of 21, as well as vision and hearing, developmental assessments and body mass index (BMI) screenings for obesity
- Mammograms for women over age 40
- Pap smears for cervical cancer prevention
- Colon cancer screening tests for adults over age 50

Will I Be Able to Get the Preventive Services Promised Me? Probably not. Providing preventive care takes time, and most primary care physicians already have their hands full. Ask yourself this question: The last time you were in a doctor's office, did you observe a lot of idle resources? Were doctors and nurses standing around with nothing to do? If the answer is "no," your experience is not unique. Nationwide, more than one out of every five people lives in an officially designated Health Professional Shortage Area (HPSA), and the shortage of primary-care physicians is expected to grow worse in future years.[124]

A study published in the *American Journal of Public Health* calculated how much time it would take physicians to arrange for and counsel patients about all the screening tests recommended by the U.S. Preventive Services Task Force.[125] The bad news: It would require 1,773 hours of your doctor's time each year, or 7.4 hours per working day. And all of this time is spent searching for problems and talking about the search. If the screenings turn up a real problem, more testing and more counseling must take place. The unfortunate bottom line: To meet this promise nationwide, every family doctor in America would have to work full-time delivering just preventive care — leaving no time for all of the other things doctors do!

Furthermore, since preventive screenings are often reimbursed at lower rates than other services, when you call your doctor for a preventive care appointment, you may find there is a long wait. Increasing the demand for doctors without significantly increasing the supply will lead to increased rationing of their time.

Is Preventive Medicine Cost-Effective? Much rhetoric suggests that preventive care pays for itself. If a disease is caught in its early stages, treatment costs will be lower. So can wider access to preventive care lower the nation's health care costs? In general, no.

At the individual level, the old adage that an ounce of prevention is worth a pound of cure is true.[126] For the few patients who are diagnosed with a disease, preventive screenings are definitely worth the cost. But the cost of screening thousands of healthy patients in order to find one patient with a problem usually swamps any savings on patients whose diseases are diagnosed early.

In general, preventive medicine adds to health care costs, rather than reducing them.[127] Mammograms don't pay for themselves. Neither do Pap smears, or prostate cancer tests, or even general checkups for

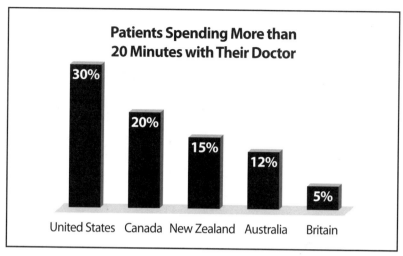

Source: Health Affairs

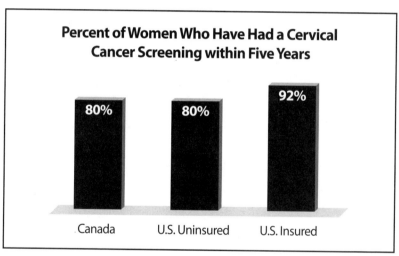

Source: Employment Policies Institute

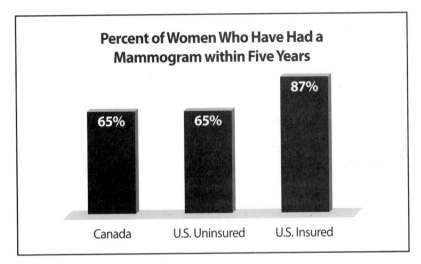

Source: Employment Policies Institute

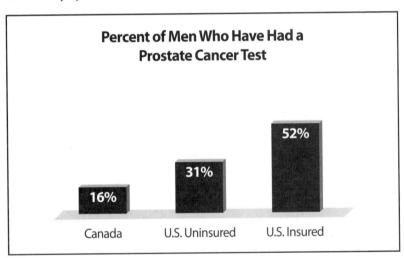

Source: Employment Policies Institute

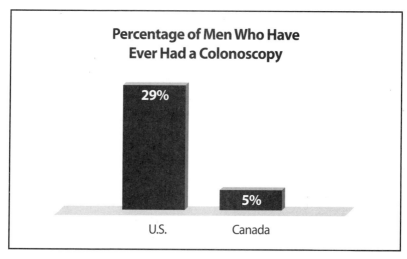

Source: National Bureau of Economic Research

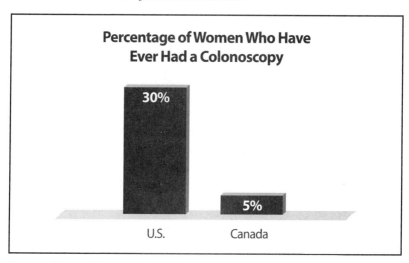

Source: National Bureau of Economic Research

healthy people. While people should not avoid preventive care, they should understand that these tests add to total spending on health care, and obtain them judiciously.

There are some exceptions — childhood immunizations and prenatal care for at-risk mothers, for example. But the exceptions are few and far between. As Louise Russell explained recently in *Health Affairs*:[128]

> Over the past four decades, hundreds of studies have shown that prevention usually adds to medical spending. [Data] from 599 studies published between 2000 and 2005 [show that] less than 20 percent of the preventive options (and a similar percentage for treatment) fall in the cost-saving category — *80 percent* add more to medical costs than they save. [Italics added.]

Can We Use Medical Science to Decide What Preventive Care People Should Get? Who should get a mammogram? At what age? How frequently? What about Pap smears and prostate cancer tests and colonoscopies? Aren't these questions experts can decide? Unfortunately, no. Any reader of daily newspapers knows that we are forever getting conflicting advice from well-meaning people. Part of the problem is that people differ in their attitude toward risk. They also differ in their willingness to spend money to reduce risk. A danger in a one-size-fits-all approach fashioned in Washington, D.C., is that government experts may not share your values. Their attitude toward risk reduction may be different from yours.

The Danger of Cookbook Medicine. Another danger is that doctors overwhelmed by far more requests for services than they can possibly deliver will take a routine approach to all their patients and ignore what makes you unique. What if you are at a heightened risk for breast cancer because your mother or grandmother had breast cancer — but you fall outside the guidelines for early breast cancer screening before age 40? Susan G. Komen Race for the Cure recommends that women at higher risk of breast cancer begin testing at age 25.[129] But will you be allowed to do so? Even if you pay for the test yourself? We don't yet know.

The Dangers of the Politics of Medicine. Both Congress and the administration have already shown that they are unwilling to let experts set the guidelines for preventive care. For example, the new law stipulates that seniors are entitled to an annual physical and that males are entitled to an annual prostate cancer test — even though the Preventive Services Task Force recommends neither. Also, Health and Human Services Secretary Sebelius has chosen to include annual mammograms for women in their 40s, even though the task force recommended against it.

Also, while more "free" services may sound good, remember that the doctor's time is limited, as are the number of health care dollars. Granting more marginal care to one person may mean less really serious care for another.

Letting Individuals Make Their Own Choices. There is a better way. Instead of one-size-fits-all medicine, individuals can make many of their own choices in these matters. Instead of giving all of your health care dollars to an impersonal, bureaucratic insurance company, you should be allowed to put some of those dollars in a health savings account that you own and control.[130] Thus, you could consult the advice of the Preventive Services Task Force on your own. You could also consider the advice of other experts, including your doctor, and take into consideration personal data about you and your family.

Ultimately, no one cares about you more than you. If you control more of the money and are allowed to make more of your own decisions, the system is likely to work better for you than if you cede that power and control to others.

Preventive care is not like an *investment good* that pays a positive rate of return. Instead, it's like a *consumption good*. Preventive care leads to better health. But the enjoyment of that result must be compared with the benefit of other goods and services we could have purchased with the same money.

What About Contraception?

The federal health care law classifies contraception as a preventive service. Beginning in 2012, the law requires health insurance purchased by an employer and sold in the exchange to cover contraception without cost sharing.[131] Grandfathered plans, and certain religious institutions that oppose contraception, are exempt from this mandate.[132]

More than 45 lawsuits have been filed by organizations opposed to this controversial mandate, mainly because contraceptives include "morning after" pills, which many of these groups consider a form of abortion.[133] Under ObamaCare, houses of worships are also exempt from the contraception mandate, but nonprofit religious-affiliated groups are not.[134] This issue appears to be headed to the Supreme Court.[135]

What About Abortion?

The Hyde Amendment prohibits using federal dollars to directly fund abortions. However, the law does allow federal monies to provide coverage for abortions due to rape, incest or life-threatening pregnancies.[136] And insurers are permitted to include abortion coverage through the state-based exchanges when people purchase the private insurance with a combination of personal money and federal subsidy. However, to ensure that no subsidy dollars are directed toward these purposes, consumers who purchase insurance that covers abortion (whether that is their specific goal or not) will be required to make two premium payments — one to cover abortion services and one to cover everything else.[137] The federal subsidy can be used only to defray the cost of the latter.[138]

Pro-life groups claim this two-payment system is nothing more than an accounting gimmick. They say the federal government will in effect be funding abortions unless all federally subsidized individuals are prevented from choosing insurance plans that cover abortion. Abortion rights advocates also complain that few states will offer plans that cover abortion due to the cumbersome two-payment system. Their concerns are warranted as the law not only allows state exchanges to prohibit plans that offer abortion coverage, it allows states to pass laws prohibiting abortion coverage by exchanges. Since 2010, five states have already done this.[139]

Are Electronic Medical Records Safe, Effective and Private?

Doctors who see Medicare and Medicaid patients will face financial penalties if they fail to adopt electronic medical records (EMRs), under the 2009 federal stimulus bill. This is the first step the government has taken toward a goal of universal EMRs by 2014, although the system is behind schedule.

When you visit your doctor, a record of the visit will be stored electronically. The record will contain all of the information exchanged between you and your doctor, your doctor's notes, any drug prescriptions you receive and any disease prognosis you are given. Your EMR will even contain a government-approved obesity rating — a body mass index measuring your body fat percentage. These obesity ratings will be sent automatically to federal health agencies such as the Department of Health and Human Services and the Centers for Disease Control. The government also aims to make sure your EMR is compatible with other records and kept in a format that can be accessed by other doctors and hospital personnel, regardless of where you seek care.

Is this a good idea?

Will EMRs Improve the Quality of My Care? Maybe. Or maybe not. Formal evaluations are generally lacking, and the jury is still out. Potentially, EMRs could enhance the coordination of care among diverse doctors and hospitals. Providers could see which tests you have already undergone and their results, thereby saving you the money and inconvenience of duplicate tests. Medical personnel would also learn what prescription drugs you are taking, any drug allergies you may have and other vital information. Ideally this information should allow doctors to deliver safer and more effective care. On the other hand, if your EMR is not properly maintained, doctors could make serious mistakes that could be hazardous to your health. For example:[140]

- In one case, a mother of three died of cancer after going untreated for three to six months because the report from her radiologist was not filed properly in her EMR, leaving her referring physician completely unaware of her condition.
- Another lab test result, improperly filed in a patient's EMR, ultimately caused the patient to suffer from acute renal failure.
- Records entered into the wrong EMR left another patient untreated for congestive heart failure, from which he later died.
- A woman's baby was born brain dead due to umbilical strangulation and later died when her obstetrician, monitoring the baby's birth from his home using the patient's EMR, was unaware of software glitches that concealed vital patient information.
- In another case, three days passed before a patient's care team realized the results entered into his EMR were for a biopsy they did not order of a lesion the patient did not have.

These mistakes are more common than you might suppose. More than 200 adverse events associated with EMRs have been reported to the Food and Drug Administration in the past two years.[141]

Another problem is information overload. The time your doctor spends entering your data can detract from your care. A doctor struggling to enter patient information into multiple screens—each with multiple check boxes — could miss subtle clues that might have been observed if he or she were interacting with you face-to-face. Furthermore, some EMRs automatically generate redundant information that can clutter a record containing important medical problems or create false-alarm alerts for minor drug interactions.

Will EMRs Save Money? Two highly influential studies by the RAND Corporation[142] and the Center for Information Technology Leadership[143] estimated health information technology—including EMRs — could potentially save $77 billion to $78 billion per year if adopted by virtually all doctors and hospitals. However, most doctors and most hospitals find that the adoption of EMRs adds to their costs rather than reduces them.[144] Thus, as with the question of quality, the jury is still out.

How Well Are EMRs Working Where They Have Been Adopted? That depends. EMR systems seem to work well where they have been voluntarily chosen by doctors trying to solve their own information flow problems. They do not seem to work well when they are imposed top-down, against the doctors' wishes.[145]

The British experience with EMRs has been disappointing.[146] While the Obama administration is in the process of spending billions on developing EMRs, the British government has concluded that its £12.7 billion national EMR system is a failure and that "there can be no confidence that the programme has delivered or can be delivered as originally conceived." In a report on this information technology (IT) program, the *Telegraph (U.K.)* quoted Andrew Lansley, the Health Secretary, as saying, "Labour's NHS IT Programme let down the NHS and wasted taxpayers' money by imposing a top-down IT system on the local NHS, which didn't fit their needs."[147]

Will My Privacy Be Protected? Some of the information in your EMR may be potentially embarrassing. It could also be used against you — say, by an employer trying to avoid workers with costly health conditions, or even by an unfriendly coworker. No matter how much effort is made to secure the records, EMRs always entail a risk to patient privacy. Hospital or medical office employees, for example, have been known to steal electronic medical records. And EMRs will always be susceptible to hackers motivated by voyeurism or even outright blackmail — to steal personal information in order to cash in by making false claims.

- A California Health Department investigation of incidents of patient "snooping" at the UCLA Medical Center found that over a five-year period more than 100 hospital workers had inappropriately viewed the records of 1,041 patients — including then-California First Lady Maria Shriver.[148]
- Actress Farrah Fawcett's EMR was hacked while she was undergoing treatment for cancer, resulting in details of her treatment being made available to the public.[149]

- After Dallas Cowboys Pro Bowl defensive tackle Erik Williams suffered a season-ending knee injury in a car accident, his electronic records were viewed online by 1,754 separate Parkland Hospital employees.[150] Less than a few dozen people had a medical reason to view them.
- In Britain, computer hackers were able to obtain the medical records of British Prime Minister Gordon Brown.[151]

What About Identity Theft? New revelations raise the specter of identity theft. Websites that store sensitive data must be designed to withstand all threats that could compromise the security of their data. But as we have seen, this (at least initially) was not considered in designing the HealthCare.gov website. Some experts say it could take a year to reduce risks to personal information.[152] In some cases, it may be impossible to mitigate all threats to security.

Electronic medical records make this cyber-crime much easier. In 2006, an individual whose cousin provided him with the EMRs of 1,100 Medicare patients from a clinic where he worked made $2.8 million in fraudulent claims.[153] The federal government reported more than 250,000 incidents of medical identity theft in 2007 alone.[154] The real number of victims is probably much higher, however. Most patients are unaware of any misdeed until they see their credit report or are informed by their insurance company that their lifetime cap on benefits has been reached. This is especially risky on HealthCare.gov because the law does not require the federal government to announce any cases of identity theft.[155] The state exchanges are required to report any security breaches, but the federal exchange is released from that obligation, meaning tthat millions of dollar's worth of information could be taken without the public knowing it.

What Will Happen to My Taxes?

You will join other Americans in paying more than $500 billion in 19 new types of taxes and fees over the next decade to fund health reform.[156] You will pay some of the taxes indirectly, in the form of higher prices, higher premiums or lower wages. You will pay others directly. According to the Joint Committee on Taxation, about 73 million taxpayers earning less than $200,000 will see their taxes rise as a result of various health reform provisions.[157]

Tax on Medical Devices. These taxes apply to everything from surgical instruments and bedpans to wheelchairs and crutches. Even pacemakers and artificial hips and knees are taxed, as well as such drugstore items as bandages and toothbrushes. All told, the tax on medical devices will collect nearly $20 billion over the next decade.

Tax on Insurance. A $60 billion tax on health insurance that began in 2014 will ultimately be reflected in higher premiums. For example, the Finance Committee's Republican staff estimates the new taxes — including taxes on medical devices, taxes on drugs, taxes on insurers — could ultimately push up health insurance premiums for a typical family of four by nearly $1,000 per year.[158]

Tax on Drugs. The new tax on drugs that began in 2011 will collect about $27 billion through 2019.[159] These taxes and the changes in the treatment of medical savings accounts (described below) have been called the "medicine cabinet tax."

Tax on Medical Savings Accounts. As of January 1, 2011, if you have a flexible spending account (FSA), a health reimbursement arrangement (HRA) or a health savings account (HSA), you may no longer use these tax-free accounts to purchase over-the-counter drugs. That means you will have to buy such items as Claritin, aspirin or Advil with after-tax dollars — making the cost to you 30 percent higher or more. In addition, tax-free contributions to an FSA will be capped at $2,500 annually. People setting aside funds for chronic care, corrective eye surgery or other out-of-pocket medical expenses will be limited to $2,500 annually, regardless of medical need. Taken together, these two actions are expected to cost consumers $18 billion over the next decade.

Taxes on Indoor Tanning. If you plan to use an indoor tanning bed, expect to pay 10 percent more thanks to a new excise tax expected to raise nearly $3 billion.

Taxes on Cadillac Plans. A 40 percent excise tax will be levied on so-called "Cadillac" health plans that provide enrollees with a benefit package worth more than $27,500 for families and $10,200 for single coverage. Beginning in 2019, the tax will impact about one-third of health plans. But these thresholds are not designed to increase as medical costs rise, therefore the tax will eventually affect all plans.

Taxes on Illness. If you have high medical expenses, today's tax law allows you to deduct from your taxable income the amount that exceeds a certain level of your adjusted gross income (AGI). In 2013, this threshold was increased from 7.5 to 10 percent of AGI — making your deduction smaller.

Additional Taxes on Wages, Investment Income and Home Sales. In 2013, the Medicare payroll tax increased by almost one-third for individuals and couples — from 2.9 to 3.8 percent on wages over $200,000 for an individual or $250,000 for a couple. In addition, the 3.8 percent Medicare payroll tax will be levied on investment income (capital gains, interest and dividend income) at the same income levels. This tax will not merely reach the rich, however. Under some circumstances, the sale of a house could trigger the provision, making you "paper rich" for a single year, forcing you to pay a 3.8 percent levy on a portion of your home's appreciated value above a certain limit. Moreover, the threshold above which people must pay the higher tax is not indexed to rise with inflation. Consequently, over time, more and more middle-class Americans will have to pay it.

What If I Am on Medicare?

The new health reform law is likely to affect Medicare enrollees more than any other population group.

Benefits of Reform. There are a number of new benefits, including:

- Medicare is paying for an annual wellness exam.

- Deductibles and copayments for many preventive services and screenings (colonoscopies, mammograms, bone mass density tests and so forth) have been eliminated.
- Eventually (in 2019), the "doughnut hole" in prescription coverage will be eliminated.

Meeting the Promises of Reform. How do you know that when you and millions of elderly and disabled patients try to get your free annual wellness exam, mammogram or colonoscopy, there will be enough doctors, nurses, laboratories and testing equipment to supply these new services? You don't. Unfortunately, the new health reform law does not provide the funding needed to make sure these promises can be kept. If everyone on Medicare took advantage of a free annual wellness exam, for example, we would need 23,000 additional doctors just to meet the demand. [See "What About Preventive Care?"]

Costs of Reform. Reduced Medicare spending, amounting to $715 billion over the next 10 years, will pay for more than half the cost of health reform:[160]

- Cuts to hospital services total $260 billion.
- Cuts to Medicare Advantage Plans total $156 billion.
- Cuts to skilled nursing, hospice, home health and other services add up to $155 billion.
- Hospitals that treat a disproportionate share of indigent patients will lose $56 billion.

The elderly and disabled will incur significant costs:

- In general, the Medicare spending cuts exceed the new benefits by a factor of more than 10 to 1.[161]
- As a result, one of every two people expected to participate in Medicare Advantage over the next 10 years (7.4 million of 14 million) will lose their coverage entirely. According to Medicare's chief actuary, they will be tossed back into Medicare, with the option to buy another Advantage plan or a supplement; and those who retain their Advantage coverage will face steep benefit cuts or hefty premium increases, or both.[162]

- Additionally, indirect costs, including new taxes on drugs and medical devices — will apply to items that are disproportionately used by seniors and the disabled.

To make matters worse, Medicare's chief actuary believes the planned cuts in fees may cause some doctors to retire and force some hospitals out of business.[163] Moreover, as 100 million newly and more generously insured people try to increase their consumption of medical care, you may find it increasingly difficult to obtain the care you need.

Coverage for Prescription Drugs. Seniors who have retiree drug coverage through their employer are at risk of losing that coverage. Provisions of the Affordable Care Act have caused employers to eliminate the plans of more than 3 million beneficiaries — forcing them to choose new plans, with possible changes in premiums and copayments.[164] Previously, employers who provided their employees with postretirement health care benefits could set up and administer retiree drug plans as an alternative to Medicare Part D. In return, employers got subsidies worth about $665 per retiree, and tax breaks made the value of the subsidy even higher. The health reform law repealed the tax subsidy, however. The loss to major employers is substantial:[165]

- AT&T estimates the change will cost it $1 billion.
- John Deere estimates it stands to lose $150 million.
- Caterpillar puts the loss at $100 million.
- A Credit Suisse report estimates that S&P 500 companies face losses of $4.5 billion.

In response, many large firms will completely eliminate their retiree drug plans.

In addition, 27 million seniors will pay higher premiums for the Medicare Part D Plan in order to close the doughnut hole. An estimated 4 million seniors reach the doughnut hole annually, but fewer than 1 million will surpass the threshold and receive the full benefit of closing the doughnut hole. Expect your premiums to rise 9 percent in 2019 as a result.[166]

Size of the Cuts in Medicare Spending. The table below lists the expected spending reductions for Medicare enrollees. If you are in conventional Medicare, you can expect that reduced spending to average $290 this year. If you are in a Medicare Advantage plan, you can expect more severe cuts: $1,267 in 2014. If you are able to retain your coverage, these cuts will lead to increases in premiums or reductions in benefits, or both.

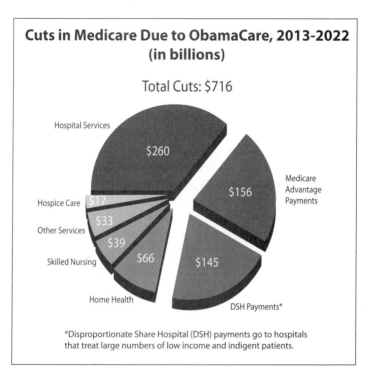

Cuts in Medicare Due to ObamaCare, 2013-2022 (in billions)

Total Cuts: $716

Hospital Services $260
Medicare Advantage Payments $156
Hospice Care $17
Other Services $33
Skilled Nursing $39
Home Health $66
DSH Payments* $145

*Disproportionate Share Hospital (DSH) payments go to hospitals that treat large numbers of low income and indigent patients.

Source: Heritage Foundation

Some of the early reductions required by federal law have been delayed in the interest of disrupting seniors' health plan choices as little as possible. For instance, in 2012, the administration established an $8.35 billion demonstration program to reward Medicare Advantage plans exhibiting high-quality standards.[167] Many experts believe this was a carrot designed to delay the painful cuts to Medicare Advantage plans until after the 2012 election. The last thing the administration wanted was for millions of seniors to lose their coverage just before an election. In 2013, a planned 2.2

percent subsidy decrease was replaced with a 3.3 percent increase.[168] This delay was also the result of lobbying by members of Congress, insurers and advocates for seniors.

Note that these delayed cuts are on top of a planned 25 percent cut in Medicare physician fees pursuant to a pre-existing law, which Congress has been postponing for the past seven years.

Comparing the path we have been on to the path required under the new law:[169]

- The annual reduction in spending will reach $2,300 per beneficiary by 2020, $3,844 by 2030 and $9,413 by midcentury (all numbers at current prices).
- By the time today's teenagers reach retirement age, *one-third of Medicare will effectively be gone.*

The Obama administration claims that it will target these cuts to eliminate waste — to encourage low-cost, high-quality care and discourage high-cost, low-quality practices. But critics are not hopeful. In fact, Medicare's own actuaries believe that spending cuts will most likely be made through reductions in fees paid to doctors, hospitals and other providers. As is reflected in the chart below, private insurers already pay fees far more generous than Medicare or Medicaid. If Medicare cuts go through as planned, by the end of this decade, the Medicare fees paid to physicians will fall to about half private insurers' fees — and well below the paltry fees that Medicaid pays physicians.

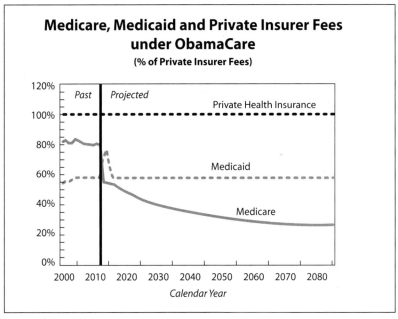

Medicare, Medicaid and Private Insurer Fees under ObamaCare

(% of Private Insurer Fees)

Source: U.S. Department of Health and Human Services

- Medicare fees will fall below Medicaid rates by 2019 and continue to fall further behind other payers in the years that follow.
- By 2050, Medicare will pay only half as much as private plans pay; by 2080, it will pay only one-third.

These cuts are so draconian that the Medicare actuaries warn that doctors will be unwilling to see Medicare patients, and hospitals and other facilities will be forced to leave the Medicare program. Overall, the actuaries predict that:[170]

- By 2019, one in seven facilities will become unprofitable and will probably be forced to leave the Medicare program.
- That number will grow to 25 percent of all facilities by 2030 and to 40 percent by 2050.

How Cuts in Medicare Spending Will Be Made. The new law assumes that the federal government can make Medicare grow at about half the rate of growth of health care spending overall and eventually no faster than the rate of growth of national income. To achieve this goal, the law gives an Independent Payment Advisory Board (IPAB) the power to adopt more Medicare spending cuts. Congress must either accept these cuts or propose its own plan to cut costs as much or more than the IPAB's proposal. If Congress fails to substitute its own plan, the IPAB's cuts will become effective. Thus, the growth rate of Medicare spending is officially capped.

This approach gives an independent agency much more power than any similar agency has had before. However, there are two problems. First, the IPAB is barred from considering just about any cost control idea other than cutting fees to doctors, hospitals and other suppliers. Second, these limits imply that Medicare fees will fall further and further behind private payments, making Medicare patients less desirable customers to the medical community. In some parts of the country, doctors have already become reluctant to take Medicare patients[171] — a Mayo primary care clinic in Arizona, for example, has made this decision.[172] In the not-too-distant future, Medicare patients could find themselves in the same position as Medicaid enrollees — who often are forced to get all their care at community health centers and the emergency rooms of safety net hospitals.[173] Ultimately, if Medicare spending grows at a lower rate than the health care system as a whole, the elderly and the disabled will end up in a completely different health care system. You will not be able to see the same doctors, enter the same hospitals or get the same quality of care that other Americans can.

Do Medicare Advantage Plans Deserve a Smaller Subsidy?
Critics of the program argue that the government is paying these plans about 13 percent more than what enrollees would cost if they were in conventional Medicare. While that appears to be true, let's look at the other side of the story:

- Part of the overpayment is due to Congress's desire to make Medicare Advantage plans available in rural areas, where they are less economical.

- Elsewhere, overpayments (such as extra coverage for drugs) are creating benefits for enrollees of up to $825 per year.[174]

- Even as Congress cuts Advantage plan payments, it is expanding drug coverage for Medicare enrollees — indicating that the pressure to provide the benefits will remain after the Advantage plans are gone.

- Enrollees tend to be moderate-income seniors who do not have Medigap insurance; thus, Medicare Advantage coverage is solving a social problem that will have to be solved in some other way if this program cannot.[175]

- And if millions of seniors go from Advantage plans back into conventional Medicare, paying discounted rates to providers, all seniors may find access to care more difficult.

Moreover, the Medicare Advantage plans that are headed for extinction are ostensibly doing many of the things President Obama says he wants to accomplish with health reform:[176]

- They provide subsidized coverage to low-and moderate-income people who could otherwise not afford it.

- They control costs better than conventional insurance by eliminating unnecessary care.

- They provide higher-quality care.

- They have no pre-existing condition limitations, and some plans actually specialize in attracting and caring for patients with multiple illnesses.

- They provide an annual choice of plans.

- They compete against a public plan (conventional Medicare).

What About the Medicare Trust Fund? Department of Health and Human Services Secretary Kathleen Sebelius has claimed that cuts in Medicare spending will help Medicare's Trust Fund, making it easier to pay benefits in future years.[177] Yet CBO Director Douglas W. Elmendorf rejected such claims, saying that they amount to "double-counting."[178] Either the money that is saved by cuts in Medicare spending (a) will be used to pay for health insurance for younger people or (b) will be put aside to pay

Medicare benefits in the future. But you cannot use the same dollars to buy two different things. Since the law explicitly uses cuts in Medicare spending to finance health insurance subsidies for young people, it does nothing to aid the future financial health of Medicare. Medicare's chief actuary has said the same thing.[179]

In fact, differences within the Obama administration led to a series of unprecedented events connected to the release of the Medicare Trustees report. In August 2010, several days in advance of the 2010 report, Secretary Sebelius released details favorable to the administration — including the claim that health reform would extend the life of the Medicare Trust fund by 12 years.[180] Then, when the report itself was released, Richard Foster, Medicare's chief actuary, appended a note disavowing it, encouraging readers to ignore it and drawing attention to an "alternative report" with entirely different conclusions. The Medicare actuaries' alternative report argued the assumptions underlying the projections in the Trustees' Report were "unreasonable" and "implausible" and unlikely to occur.

Unfunded Obligations of Social Security and Medicare*

	Unfunded Obligations through Infinite Horizon (2013)	Unfunded Obligations through Infinite Horizon (2012)	Change from 2012 to 2013
OASDI (Social Security)	$ 25.8 trillion	$ 23.1 trillion	+2.7
Medicare	$43.1 trillion	$ 43.1 trillion	0.0
Total Medicare and Social Security	$68.9 trillion	$ 66.2 trillion	+2.7

*This ignores the existence of the OASDI and HI trust funds, valued at 2.7 trillion, since these funds do not add real assets.

Source: 2013 Medicare Trustees Report

What about Andy Griffith? At a cost to the taxpayers of about $708,000, a television ad featured the late Andy Griffith telling viewers how great the new health law will be. Yet a fact-check by the Annenberg Public Policy Center found the claim not believable:

> Currently, about 1 in every 4 Medicare beneficiaries is enrolled in a Medicare Advantage plan. For many of them, the words in this ad ring hollow, and the promise that "benefits will remain the same" is just as fictional as the town of Mayberry was when Griffith played the local sheriff.[181]

What About AARP? The organization that claims to represent seniors has been fully supportive of the new law. But the interest of AARP and the interest of seniors are not the same. Why? AARP markets its own Medigap insurance, collecting more in premiums and revenue from other commercial ventures than it collects in member dues. With fewer seniors in MA plans, the market for Medigap insurance will greatly expand. Moreover, AARP is getting special treatment under health reform. Specifically, AARP's Medigap insurance is exempt from:[182]

- The prohibition on pre-existing condition exclusions.
- A $500,000 cap on executive compensation for insurance industry executives.
- The tax on insurance companies.
- A requirement imposed on MA plans to spend at least 85 percent of their premium dollars on medical claims.

What If I Have to Be in Medicaid?

As ObamaCare begins to take effect, millions of Americans will find themselves with no health insurance options. If you are under 65 years of age, your income is less than 139 percent of the federal poverty level and you do not have employer coverage, you must enroll in Medicaid if it is available in your state. In fact, nearly half of the newly insured under the health care reform are headed for Medicaid — many losing their private coverage in the process.

There are a few exceptions. In June 2012, the Supreme Court ruled that states that decided against expanding Medicaid eligibility cannot be penalized with the loss of federal matching funds. Since then, almost half the states have decided not to expand Medicaid. As a result, some individuals earning just above the poverty line will be able to enroll in highly subsidized private coverage — with benefits that may be far better than Medicaid.[183]

However, a quirk in the law means that people with incomes below the poverty level will not be able to enter the exchange. If they are not eligible for Medicaid either, these families will have no access to subsidized insurance. And this "catch-22" glitch apparently applies to about 6.6 million people living under the poverty level who reside in states that decided not to expand their Medicaid programs.[184]

State Medicaid Expansion

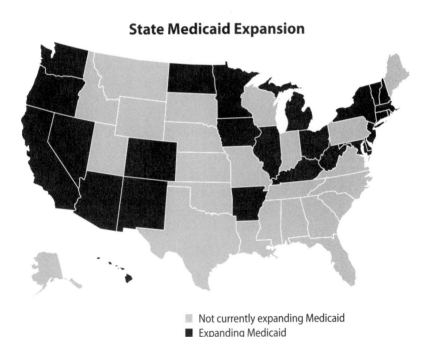

    ☐ Not currently expanding Medicaid
    ■ Expanding Medicaid

Source: Kaiser Family Foundation

Worse Access to Care. Medicaid is certainly attractive on paper. Participants are promised coverage for most medical services, with no premium and usually no out-of-pocket payments. But Medicaid pays physicians only about 60 percent as much as private insurers pay, and many Medicaid patients have difficulty finding doctors who will see them. Studies show that even the uninsured have an easier time making doctors' appointments than Medicaid enrollees.[185] One survey finds that:[186]

- In Dallas and Philadelphia, only 8 percent of cardiologists accept Medicaid patients; in Los Angeles, it's 11 percent.

- In both Dallas and New York City, only 14 percent of obstetrician/gynecology specialists will see Medicaid patients; the figure is 28 percent in Miami and 33 percent in Denver.

- Among general practitioners, the lowest figures are 30 percent (Los Angeles), 40 percent (Miami) and 50 percent (Dallas and Houston).

These numbers may indicate why Medicaid enrollees seek care in the emergency room twice as often as patients covered by private plans.[187] Emergency room visits are likely to increase in the future as millions of people swell Medicaid's rolls.

Worse Health Outcomes. Numerous studies have found that Medicaid enrollees fare worse than patients with private insurance and even worse than patients with no insurance at all![188] For example:

- A University of Virginia study found that compared to the privately insured, individuals enrolled in Medicaid are almost twice as likely to die after surgery, and they are about one-eighth more likely to die than the uninsured.[189]

- A study published in the *Journal of the National Cancer Institute* found that, compared to the uninsured, Florida Medicaid patients were 6 percent more likely to be diagnosed with prostate cancer at less treatable, later stages. Medicaid enrollees were nearly one-third (31 percent) more likely to be diagnosed with late-stage breast cancer and 81 percent more likely to be diagnosed with melanoma at a late stage. (Medicaid patients were, however, less likely than the uninsured to be diagnosed with late-stage colon cancer.)[190]

- A study in the journal Cancer found that the mortality rate for Medicaid patients undergoing colon cancer surgery was over three times higher than for the privately insured and more than one-fourth higher than for the uninsured.[191]

- A study in the *Journal of Vascular Surgery* found that Medicaid patients treated for vascular problems — including plaque in their carotid (neck) arteries, which pump blood to the brain, and obstructions in the blood vessels in their legs — fared worse than the uninsured (however, the uninsured with abdominal aneurysms fared worse than Medicaid patients).[192]

Though these results have been somewhat disputed, the state of Oregon has provided fodder for a gold standard test. The state lacked sufficient funds to expand Medicaid eligibility to everyone, so in 2008 Oregon used a lottery to select about 30,000 would-be Medicaid recipients.[193] However, a report published in the *New England Journal of Medicine* found that (as far as physical health is concerned) the new Medicaid enrollees' health status was no better than those who were not selected.[194] New Medicaid enrollees reported more doctor visits and positive feelings about their coverage, but their doctors couldn't detect significant improvements in health status. Some proponents of Medicaid expansion argue that the study may have failed to show significant effects because there were too few people in each disease category.[195]

New Payment Rates. The federal government was supposed to increase Medicaid reimbursement rates to Medicare levels (80 percent of what private insurers pay) for primary care physicians in 2013 and 2014. However, most doctors have yet to see any additional payments. And while this change is designed to improve access to primary care services, it will do nothing to improve access to specialists! Moreover, in 2015, states may lower their payment rates for primary care back to the original levels — a likely outcome considering that many states will face large budgetary problems precisely because of Medicaid expansion.

What If I Have a Health Savings Account?

If you are one of more than 30 million people enrolled in a health savings account (HSA) or a health reimbursement arrangement (HRA), or if you work for the one of every two employers who now offer one of these consumer-driven health plans, in the future you will have fewer options. The new health care law does not outlaw HSA-eligible plans, but it limits HSA options, and future regulations could make these plans impractical and undesirable.

How Health Savings Accounts Work. Instead of giving all of your health care dollars to an insurance company, the current law allows you to choose a plan with a high deductible and more limited benefits, with the resulting premium savings going into an account you own and control. Deposits to these accounts may be made with pretax dollars, the same as employer-paid premiums, and the accounts grow tax-free. Because you get to keep the money you don't spend, this self-insuring allows you to directly benefit from being a prudent consumer in the medical marketplace.

Lower Deductibles. The new law reduces the allowed deductible for small-group plans (those with fewer than 100 employees) to $2,000 for singles and $4,000 for families, beginning in 2014. This is roughly one-third the level allowed under current HSA law. This will limit your ability to save on insurance premiums by joining a higher deductible plan.[196]

Larger Penalties. If you take money out of your HSA for a nonmedical purpose, the law increases the penalty from 10 to 20 percent, and you will have to pay ordinary income taxes as well. In addition, patients may not use their HSA funds to purchase over-the-counter drugs. This requirement is now especially unfortunate, because off-patent drugs typically become less expensive.

Additional Risks. The Department of Health and Human Services has the authority to review health plan benefits on an annual basis and determine the "essential" benefits that should be included in all health plans. If the Department determines that all plans must have a benefit that violates the regulations for HSA-eligibility, HSAs could essentially be outlawed by the stroke of a (regulatory) pen. Although this appears unlikely at the moment, advocates for increased consumer involvement in health care worry.[197]

Other restrictions could make HSA plans impractical. For example, critics have proposed that employers verify that every single HSA withdrawal is for medical care. This obligation would greatly increase the administration costs of these accounts.

What If I Have a Flexible Spending Account?

The ACA has made a significant change to flexible spending accounts (FSA), by sharply reducing the annual contribution limit. Estimates vary, but about 30 million people are using FSAs. These accounts pay for such things as medical expenses, dental insurance premiums, long-term care and child care with pretax dollars. Funds must be used in the year they are set aside, however.

FSA Changes: One Good and Two Bad. Although most employers limit the amount you can contribute to $5,000, the new law will limit contributions to no more than $2,500 a year — indexed to inflation for future years.

The impact may be greater if you are one of the millions of people who use these accounts for long-term care for family members with chronic illnesses. For example, families raising special needs children often deposit funds into an FSA to pay for costly education and behavior therapy. This allows them to use pretax dollars — at a savings of nearly 50 percent in some cases — to pay for tuition that can top $1,000 per month.

The new law also changes the definition of a "qualified medical expense," prohibiting the use of funds from an FSA to pay for over-the-counter medications and products. Virtually everything in your medicine cabinet that was tax free prior to 2011 (through an FSA) is taxable. The list includes aspirin, bandages, cough syrup, cold medications, antibiotic ointment, first aid creams, pain relievers, cough drops, antacids, sinus medications, allergy medications and nasal sprays. If you are one of millions of people with a chronic condition, your costs could increase substantially.[198]

What If I Am Young?

Like all other individuals, you will be required by federal law to purchase health insurance with the specific benefits the federal government says you must have, regardless of whether you want them or whether they are useful. For instance, young single males will be required to purchase a plan that includes maternity benefits and well-baby coverage.

Benefits of Reform. Under current law, children are able to join or stay on their parents' plan until the age of 26, even if they have access to an employer plan of their own.[199]

Costs of Reform. If you are like most young people, you are healthier and have lower expected costs than older adults. For example, people in their 20s today typically face premiums that are only one-fifth or one-sixth as high as people in their 60s. The likelihood of ill health, and therefore the cost of health insurance, tends to rise with age, but fortunately so does income. People in their 50s and 60s typically pay higher premiums, but they also have higher incomes.

New regulations taking effect in 2014 will dramatically change, however, requiring insurers to accept all applicants at rates that are not adjusted for health status. Insurers may adjust premiums for age, but the highest premium can exceed the lowest by no more than a three to one ratio. Thus, young adults will face premiums much higher than their expected costs of benefits so that older, less healthy adults can pay premiums much lower than their expected costs.

The result: Young people will have to pay a lot more for coverage, perhaps even double or triple their current premium. For example, studies based on actual insurance claims data show:[200]

- The premium for a healthy 25-year-old in California will more than double — rising from $107 per month to $221.[201]
- The family premium for a 40-year-old husband and wife with two children in California would more rise by 42 percent — from $536 per month to $763.

- By contrast, a 60-year-old, less healthy couple living in California would see a drop in their premiums of about 41 percent — from $1,979 to $1,165.

Access to Catastrophic Plans. If you are under the age of 30, you will have access to health plans that have fewer mandated benefits than the standard plans. These plans will be allowed to have higher deductibles and higher cost-sharing, but out-of-pocket exposure will be no higher than HSA limits (currently $6,350 for an individual and $12,700 for a family). Presumably, these plans will have lower premiums, but they will not qualify for premium subsidies in the exchange. [See "Who Is Eligible for Catastrophic Insurance?"]

Does Marriage Help or Hurt?

It almost always hurts. The reason: Subsidies in the newly created health insurance exchange will treat two singles better than a married couple. Suppose you are earning 200 percent of the federal poverty level (currently $22,980). You will be required to pay a premium equal to 6.3 percent of your income in the exchange — or about $1,448 for a health plan that has an actual cost of, say, $5,000. Thus, you and a cohabitating partner who also earns 200 percent of the federal poverty level could both obtain health coverage for about $2,895. However, if you marry your partner, your combined income will approach 300 percent of the federal poverty level and the two of you will be required to pay 9.5 percent of your income in premiums — or about $4,366. Being married will cost the two of you $1,471 a year. For older cohabitating couples whose individual incomes are slightly below 400 percent of poverty ($62,040), the difference between getting married and cohabitating could determine whether they get a subsidy worth thousands of dollars or no subsidy at all.

In some cases, getting married may be worth the financial penalty, however. If you and your partner each earn 100 percent of the federal poverty level (currently $11,490), you would (individually) qualify for Medicaid and ineligible for private coverage in the exchange. However, if you are married, your combined income would disqualify you for Medicaid. If you bought insurance in the exchange, you would be required to pay 4 percent of your household income (or $919). The ability to get out of Medicaid (which pays low doctor fees) and into a private plan (which pays market rates) may be worth the extra premium — especially if you value more ready access to care.

What If I Am an Employer?

Here is the most important thing to know: Above-average wage workers get little or no subsidy in the exchange. But because premiums at work are paid with pre-tax dollars, people in higher tax brackets get substantial tax relief from employer-provided insurance — a subsidy equal to as much as half the cost of the insurance. So these employees may obtain insurance cheaper at work than they can through an exchange. And that advantage increases if the exchange in your state attracts a disproportionate number of high-cost patients, pushing up the community-rated premiums.

The opposite is true for below-average wage employees. Someone who makes too little to pay income taxes is avoiding only the payroll tax when the employer pays the premium. The subsidies are much larger in the exchanges. Your employees will be able to obtain insurance in a new health insurance exchange that is cheaper (for them) than you can purchase as an employer. So both you and your employees are probably better off, in this case, if you pay higher wages instead of health insurance premiums, and send your employees to the exchange.

Take an employee with a family who is earning, say, $30,000. If you provide the government-mandated insurance at work, the cost will equal about half the employee's salary. The only subsidy is the ability to pay premiums with dollars that are not included in the taxable income of the employee. Since this employee makes too little to pay income taxes, the only tax the employee avoids is a 15.3 percent (FICA) payroll tax of about $2,811.

If this same employee enters a health insurance exchange, however, he or she will pay a premium of only $900. The government will not only pay the entire remaining premium, it will also reimburse the family for most of its out-of-pocket costs — bringing the total expected annual subsidy to about $19,400.

So, combining the employer's financial interest with the employee's, the potential gain is about $16,589, if the employee gets health insurance in the exchange rather than at the workplace. And that money could be used to pay higher wages, provide other benefits or add to company profits.

Note also, that the financial gain from sending the employee to the exchange, as opposed to employer provided insurance, in this case far exceeds a potential $2,000 fine. It also exceeds the value of any small-business health insurance tax credit, discussed below.

Consider a typical hotel. Almost everyone you see is earning about $15 to $20 an hour. The cost of family coverage is equal to between one-third and one-half of these workers' annual earnings. The goal of the health reform law is to force the employer and the employees to obtain this insurance with no extra help from government. The economic literature on this type of mandate is clear. Employee benefits are not gifts from employers. They are substitutes for money wages and other benefits. Ultimately, the employees will likely bear the cost of the employer mandate. Empirical research by economists confirms health benefits are offset dollar for dollar by lower cash wages.[202]

We can be fairly certain that low-wage workers and their employers will be searching for ways to avoid the mandate. Here are some options:

Stay small. As long as employers restrict their workforce to no more than 49 employees, the mandate doesn't apply. One perverse result is that many firms will avoid growth beyond 49 employees.[203] Warning: If you own two franchise restaurants, the IRS will count that as a single business, not as two separate businesses.

Use part-time labor. Another option is to move employees to part-time status (fewer than 30 hours a week) rather than full-time. For those who try to use part-time labor to stay under the

50-employee mark, the IRS found an answer to that strategy as well. It will count two 20-hour-a-week employees as equivalent to one full-time employee in determining how many employees the firm employs.

Even if the mandate applies, the employer does not have to offer insurance to part-timers. Some firms have already begun dropping coverage to part-timers.[204] In addition, many other firms are reducing full-time workers' hours back to part time.[205] There are more than 100 printed pages of regulations on determining what is a "full-time" employee.[206]

Use non-employee labor. Independent contractors by definition are not employees. As long as they don't work regular hours, workers can retain their contractor status even if they work at the employer's establishment. The temp business is booming in anticipation of this. Another approach is to turn employees into self-incorporated businesses. As one business owner says, "There is almost nothing that cannot be outsourced."[207]

Charge employees the maximum allowable premium. Under the new law, health insurance is deemed "affordable" if the employee's premium does not exceed 9.5 percent of the employee's wages. One way to discourage employees from accepting the employer offer of health insurance is to charge them the maximum allowable premium for individual coverage and the full cost of family coverage.

Self-insure. Larger employers can reduce costs (see below) by self-insuring, essentially acting as their own insurers and paying workers' medical claims for plans administered by a third-party administrator. More than half the workers in the country work for a self-insured employer, a trend that has grown since passage of the Affordable Care Act.[208]

Meet minimum benefits requirement by providing preventive care with no annual or lifetime limit. For a self-insured company, this action avoids the $2,000 fine per full-time employee. However, because it does not meet the required minimum value of health coverage, the employer risks a $3,000 fine if the employee goes to the exchange and obtains subsidized insurance. Still, most employees are unlikely to seek more expensive insurance unless they have a health problem. And if they do, the fine is likely to be well below the employee's cost of medical care.

Offer top-up insurance. To avoid even the possibility of a $3,000 fine, the employer can give employees the option to top up their coverage to full (ObamaCare) compliance for 9.5 percent of their wage. Note: the employer can ask the employee to pay the full cost of the dependent's coverage.

Pay the fine. Employers can drop health insurance coverage altogether (or never provide it in the first place) and pay a fine equal to $2,000 per employee. That's a stiff price to pay, but it's less than the cost of health insurance. If the employer chooses this option, the employees will be eligible for subsidized insurance in the exchange.

In all cases, coverage is deemed affordable so long as the self-only coverage does not exceed 9.5 percent of the worker's pay. Whether or not the cost of family coverage exceeds 9.5 percent of family income is irrelevant. Thus, employers are free to cut back on family coverage even though this will likely result in millions of uninsured family members who cannot afford to be on their spouse's or parents' health plan and do not qualify for subsidized exchange coverage.

What If I Run a Small Business?

Mandated Health Insurance. If your company employs fewer than 50 full-time workers, you will be exempt from penalties for failing to offer health coverage. The 50th worker, however, could be a very expensive hire. If you employ 50 or more workers, failure to provide insurance will subject you to a tax penalty of $2,000 for each uninsured employee beyond the first 30 employees. So growing from 49 to 50 uninsured workers would subject you to a fine of $40,000 [(50-30) x $2,000] for adding the last worker. This fine, however, will be much smaller than the cost of providing 50 employees with the insurance mandated under the ACA.

A Catch-22. If you are already providing insurance, you may be able to retain your current health plan by claiming grandfathered status.[209] This would make you immune from cost-increasing regulatory burdens, because the mandated benefit package is likely to be more generous and more costly than what you have now. However, very few small businesses will be able to do this.[210]

Moreover, any substantial change in your health plan, such as switching to a new insurance carrier, will cause you to lose your grandfathered status — even though small firms keep premiums down primarily by changing insurers. As a result, you can accept double-digit premium increases for your existing insurance — currently averaging 10 to 18 percent nationwide — or you can shop for new coverage, in which case you will lose your grandfathered status and have to comply with dozens of costly new mandates.

- Under a mid-range estimate, two-thirds of small-business employees will lose their grandfathered status this year and will no longer be able to keep the plan they now have.[211]
- Under the worst-case scenario, as many as 80 percent will lose their grandfathered status.[212]
- By contrast, a self-insured, large company plan or union plan is free to change its third-party administrator as often as it likes and still keep its grandfathered status.[213]

Employer Access to a SHOP Exchange. If you have fewer than 100 employees, you will be able to purchase coverage in a health insurance exchange rather than buy insurance in the small-group market. The so-called SHOP Exchange is behind schedule; the federal government has announced that implementation (in the 33 states that chose not to run their own exchange) will be delayed until 2015.[214] However, if you purchase coverage through the SHOP exchange, your employees will not be able to obtain the subsidies that individuals will receive if they are buying their own insurance. Also, just as insurers selling in the exchange may not charge premiums based on health status, that same requirement will also govern the small-group market outside the exchange. At this point, it is unclear whether there will be any financial advantage to using the SHOP exchange.

Potential Benefit: A New Small-Business Subsidy. The new law includes a health insurance tax credit that may help you purchase health insurance for your employees. However, the credit is available only for six years and only for firms that have 25 or fewer employees and pay annual wages that average less than $50,000 per employee. Moreover, most businesses will not meet the strict (and complex) criteria for claiming the credit. In fact, fewer than one-third of small businesses will qualify, according to the National Federation of Independent Business, the trade association that represents small business.[215] Also, the credit is not available to sole proprietorships and their families.

Limits on Employee Premiums. If you do decide to provide the mandated health insurance benefit to your employees, you may be required to limit the amount of premiums some employees pay to a percentage of their income. For example, health plans are considered unaffordable if workers earning less than 400 percent of the federal poverty level (about $45,960 for an individual) are required to pay a premium that is more than 9.5 percent of their income. The premium for an employee with an income of $30,000, for example, would be deemed unaffordable if the premium was any higher than $2,850. For firms with more than 49 workers, employing a worker whose premiums are unaffordable may result in a $3,000 fine.

The income that is relevant here, by the way, is the wage income you pay your employees compared to the cost of single-only employee coverage. Your employee health plan is not deemed unaffordable if the employee's share of family coverage exceeds 9.5 percent of family income, as most advocates had hoped.[216]

What If I Am an Early Retiree?

Under the current law, three public-policy barriers may stand between you and affordable health insurance:

- Although tax law allows employers to pay premiums for group insurance for active employees with untaxed dollars, employers cannot make premium contributions to the individually owned insurance of their retirees with untaxed dollars. (You must pay taxes on the employer's contribution and buy insurance with what's left over — which can double the cost of health insurance for a middle-income household.)

- Similarly, although many employees are able to pay their share of health insurance premiums using premium-only plans set up by their employers, retirees must pay their premiums with after-tax dollars.

- Although the ability to pay premiums with untaxed dollars makes employer-paid health insurance for current medical expenses more affordable, there is no easy means for employers and employees to save for future medical expenses — including postretirement — expenses.

Some employers have made promises of postretirement health care. Yet these tend to be all-or-nothing propositions. That is, employers can keep their retirees in their group insurance plan — paying with pretax dollars — or they can do nothing. It's hard to be in between. If an employer cannot afford, say, a $12,000 family plan for a retiree, the employer cannot split the difference and contribute $6,000 to the employee's individually owned insurance. Such a contribution would be treated as taxable income.

Unfortunately, the health reform law solves none of these problems. It does create new subsidies for employer-provided insurance for retirees, but these new subsidies phase out in 2014.[217] Moreover, the subsidies go not to individuals but to employers. Indeed, one of the ironies of the new health law is that the first subsidies went not to low-income, uninsured families but to General Motors, General Electric, Procter & Gamble, PepsiCo, Alcoa, Intel, Pfizer and other large companies. And because higher-income employees are more likely to have an employer promise of post-retirement care, the subsidies helped those early retirees who least needed help.

Now that these subsidies have ended, insurers — selling in the health insurance exchange — will have to accept all applicants regardless of health condition. On the plus side, the difference in premiums an insurer charges in the exchange cannot exceed three to one (rather than the more normal cost ratio of six to one). That means that young people will be overcharged so that older people can be undercharged. Another change that may affect you is the potential loss of your employer's retiree drug plan. Employers who provide their employees with post-retirement drug coverage receive subsidies worth about $665 per retiree, and tax breaks make the value of the subsidy even higher. The health reform law removes the tax subsidies, however.[218] In response, many large firms are expected to do away with their retiree drug plans. In fact, the latest Medicare Trustees report predicts that 90 percent of retirees with such plans will lose the coverage.[219]

Finally, many cities — including Chicago and other such bankrupt cities as Detroit and Stockton, California — are trying to unload their unfunded retiree obligations into the heath exchanges.[220]

What If I Am an Immigrant?

If you are a legal resident alien, you are required to obtain the same government-mandated health coverage that U.S. citizens must obtain. Legal immigrants must reside in the United States five years before they qualify for Medicaid assistance. To create a means for recent legal immigrants to obtain coverage, the Affordable Care Act granted an exception allowing legal immigrants with incomes between 100 and 138 percent of poverty to qualify for highly subsidized health coverage in the exchange. That means if you live in a state that did not expand Medicaid, you will be able to do something low-income U.S. citizens cannot do: obtain highly subsidized insurance (paying a premium, say, of ten cents on the dollar) in a health insurance exchange. If, as we expect, Medicaid insurance is lower-quality insurance, you will have access to better insurance than a U.S. citizen with the same income!

If you are an undocumented immigrant, you will not be subject to the individual insurance mandates, and you will not be fined if you fail to purchase health insurance. Nor will you be allowed to enroll in Medicaid or buy insurance in the health insurance exchange.

However, hospital emergency rooms will not be able to deny you health care if you are in need. Surprisingly, the most common argument for an individual mandate is that the uninsured should contribute to their own health care instead of getting it for free in the emergency room. U.S. citizens will be required to pay hefty fines if they do not obtain insurance, but if you are here illegally, you are exempted from this rule.

What If I Am a Doctor?

On the plus side, about 25 million uninsured people are expected to gain health coverage by 2022, more than half with private insurance. Some physicians may find they can opt to treat more privately insured patients (paying higher fees) by reducing the number of Medicaid and Medicare patients they see, along with patients in exchange plans that pay low fees.

Another plus, if you are seeing Medicaid patients: The law has provisions that raise Medicaid physician fees to Medicare levels in 2013 and 2014 for primary care (though not for specialists!). However, this simple task has proved harder than the administration anticipated, and implementation has been delayed in most states. Although enhanced Medicaid fees were supposed to be effective in January 2013, few doctors have seen an increase so far. Indeed, considering more than half of Medicaid enrollees are in managed care plans that do not pay physicians on a fee-for-service basis, it is not clear how states can increase Medicaid fees.[221] And even if implemented, the fees are likely to go back to their previous levels in 2015.

The biggest near-term uncertainty is how much Medicare will pay you. A 25 percent Medicare fee cut scheduled for 2014 (due to the Sustainable Growth Rate formula) has been repeatedly delayed.[222]

There are two caveats, however. First, if poor and elderly patients find it increasingly difficult to see doctors, the government will probably be forced to make major changes in the law — perhaps even forcing you to accept Medicaid patients and patients with subsidized plans.[223] Second, in Massachusetts, the subsidized plans sold in the health insurance exchange typically pay doctors somewhere between Medicare and Medicaid rates — far below what private insurers pay.

A new Medicare Independent Payment Advisory Board (IPAB) will have the authority to fast-track changes in Medicare payment rates in order to reduce the growth of Medicare spending.[224] As with the changes following the sustainable growth formula, future cuts in Medicare will likely target provider fees. The reason? All other methods of cost control are prohibited in the legislation. The IPAB's proposals may not "ration health care, raise revenues or Medicare beneficiary premiums, increase Medicare beneficiary cost-sharing (including deductibles, coinsurance, and copayments), or otherwise restrict benefits or modify eligibility criteria."

These spending reductions will take effect in 2015, although reductions in hospital payments will not begin until 2020. Also, the IPAB's decisions will not need congressional approval. Congress can only block the decisions, and in that case, it must substitute a plan that saves more money than the IPAB plan.

The biggest long-term uncertainty is how much Medicare will interfere with the practice of medicine. Almost certainly the Medicare payment system will be used to promote EMRs, coordinated care, managed care, integrated care and bundled care. At the extreme, you may be pushed into an ACO, which is an HMO-type practice with conditional fees based on a checklist of performance measures. You will be paid more if you conform, less if you don't conform — even if the end result is not good for patients. Expect private insurers to piggyback on Medicare's initiatives.

A new moratorium has been set on additional physician-owned specialty hospitals, despite evidence that these facilities lower costs and raise quality.[225]

Many physicians may respond to these uncertainties by retiring or abandoning independent practice and working for hospitals.[226] Already about half of all doctors work for hospitals or hospital-owned health care systems. When physicians go to work for hospitals, they tend to work fewer hours. If the past is any guide, physician productivity could fall by one-quarter — possibly more under these arrangements.[227] Those physicians who do remain in group practices will face competition from lesser trained medical professionals. One study is predicting that the number of walk-in clinics is going to double in the next few years.[228]

Can Health Reform Be Made Better?

Can the Affordable Care Act (ObamaCare) be improved? Can it be replaced with something much better? What follows is a health reform that does four remarkable things:

1. It is more progressive than ObamaCare (it involves more redistribution from higher to lower income households).

2. It provides genuine protection for people who develop a pre-existing condition.

3. It provides genuine access to care for everyone, in contrast to 30 million left uninsured under ObamaCare.

4. It is workable (primarily because the role of government is confined to setting a few simple rules of the game, leaving individual choice and the marketplace to do the heavy lifting).

If the alternative can be realized, it would seem to meet all the main goals of the Affordable Care Act without incurring its many hardships and arbitrary costs.

Here are the essential elements:

Choice. People should be able to choose a health plan that fits individual and family needs, rather than a plan designed by bureaucrats in Washington. This means no mandate. Men shouldn't have to buy maternity coverage; women shouldn't have to buy coverage for prostate cancer tests; teetotalers shouldn't have to buy substance abuse insurance, and so on. And no one should have to buy coverage for preventive procedures that health researchers have known for years are not cost-effective.

Fairness. Everyone at the same income level should get the same help from government when obtaining private insurance. If government subsidizes health insurance through refundable tax credits, the credit should be the same for everyone at the same income level. Should those credits vary by income, age, geography or other factors? There are good arguments for a variable credit. But there is an equally persuasive counterargument: simplicity. Suppose every adult receives an annual tax credit worth $2,500 and every child a credit worth $1,500. People would get this subsidy so long as they obtain credible private health insurance, no matter where they obtain it — at work, in the marketplace or in an exchange.

Many of our current problems would vanish.

Since a person's income would no longer be relevant, the exchanges would not have to link to the IRS, the Social Security Administration and other federal agencies (which is the main technical reason the exchanges aren't working). It wouldn't matter whether you were offered affordable coverage at work. It wouldn't matter whether you were eligible for Medicaid. If you show up at the exchange and buy private insurance, you get the credit. Period.

With a uniform tax credit, 90 percent of the problems the exchanges are now having would disappear. Signing up for insurance would be easy. Insurance companies and brokers could sign people up outside of the exchanges without asking privacy-invading questions about their income and assets.

Jobs. A uniform health insurance tax credit combined with the absence of a mandate would also eliminate the chaos ObamaCare is creating in the labor market. Without a government mandate, employers would no longer be reluctant to hire. They would no longer have an incentive to stay small (fewer than 50 full-time employees). Nor would they have an incentive to shift employees to part-time work. With a universal credit, they would no longer have an incentive to drop coverage for their active employees or end their post-retirement plans because of more generous subsidies available in an exchange.

Universality. There will always be some people who will turn down the offer of a tax credit. But instead of the Treasury keeping those unclaimed credits, the money should be sent to safety net institutions in the communities where the uninsured live. Uninsured patients will probably be asked to pay their medical bills. But if they cannot, the safety net institutions will have a source of cash to pay for "uncompensated care."

Under this idea, money follows people. The federal government promises a credit to every to every man, woman and child in the country. If everyone buys private insurance, the funds subsidize premiums. If they all decide to be uninsured, the funds go to safety net institutions. This is a way of ensuring universal access to health care. (Note: Waiting for care would still happen at many of these institutions, just as in Britain and Canada. But it would provide just as much access to care as other countries do.)

To further ensure universal access, we could allow everyone to buy into Medicaid — regardless of income. At the same time, we should allow everyone on Medicaid to leave the program, claim the tax credit and buy private insurance.

The tax credit numbers used above are the CBO estimates of the cost of enrolling new people in Medicaid. People who are already eligible could use their tax credit to buy in, no questions asked. However, people with higher incomes might have to pay a premium on top of their tax credit if they have higher-than-average expected costs. Health status wouldn't be considered. But age and other factors would be. And, to prevent gaming, no one would be able to move from one plan to another with a premium that is significantly below their total expected costs. (See below.)

Medicaid would be an insurer of last resort. But beyond their uniform tax credit, people who are not poor who enroll in Medicaid would not receive a subsidy. They would have to pay their own way.

Portability. In most states today, it is illegal for employers to buy what their employees most want and need — insurance that travels with them from job to job and in and out of the labor market. This policy needs to be reversed. Employers should be encouraged to provided portable insurance for their employees in the same way that 401(k) plans and employer-paid life insurance is portable. NFL football players and United Mine Workers already have portable insurance, with premiums paid by their employers. It's time to extend this opportunity to everyone else.

Patient Power. Health Savings Accounts (HSAs) and Health Reimbursement Arrangements (HRAs) are very effective ways to eliminate waste and control costs. That's why 30 million people now have these accounts. The RAND Corporation estimates that savings of up to 30 percent are possible by the use of these consumer-directed health care plans. And, ironically, ObamaCare is like to result in a large expansion of HSA-compatible plans.

Still, there is more we can do. Instead of the rigid restrictions of the current law, HSAs should be completely flexible — wrapping around any third-party insurance plan. Let the market determine the appropriate division between third-party insurance and individual self-insurance by means of a designated savings account. The private sector also needs the ability to create special accounts for the chronically ill. The Cash and Counseling program, under which the Medicaid disabled manage their own health care dollars, has already proven a highly successful model.

Real Insurance. No insurer should ever be allowed to dump its most costly enrollees onto another insurer without paying the full cost of the transfer. So if an expensive-to-treat patient moves from Plan A to Plan B, the former should compensate the latter for any above-average expected costs — just the way Medicare compensates private plans in the Medicare Advantage program. In this way, people will have real insurance to cover the occurrence of pre-existing conditions.

Paying for reform. How much would an alternative to ObamaCare cost? Starting from where we are now, it's almost a free lunch. If we take all of the current subsidies for employer-provided insurance and add all of the subsidies ObamaCare provides, we will have more than enough money for reasonable reform. In fact, we have enough money to give large companies and labor unions a choice of tax regimes: They can continue with the current system of tax subsidies, or they can switch to the tax credit system. Our bet: Very few will choose to stay in the old system.

Notes

[1] Stephen Dinan, "ObamaCare Has Been Amended or Delayed 19 Times: Study," *Washington Times*, September 11, 2013. Available at http://www.washingtontimes.com/news/2013/sep/11/study-ObamaCare-has-been-amended-delayed-19-times/.

[2] Robert Pear, "A Limit on Consumer Costs Is Delayed in Health Care Law," *New York Times*, August 12, 2013. Available at http://www.nytimes.com/2013/08/13/us/a-limit-on-consumer-costs-is-delayed-in-health-care-law.html.

[3] Louise Radnofsky, "Long-Term Care Gets the Ax," *Wall Street Journal*, October 15, 2011. Available at http://online.wsj.com/news/articles/SB10001424052970204002304576631302927789920.

[4] Ezra Klein, "The individual mandate no longer applies to people whose plans were canceled," *Washington Post*, Wonkblog, December 19, 2013. Available at http://www.washingtonpost.com/blogs/wonkblog/wp/2013/12/19/the-obama-administration-just-delayed-the-individual-mandate-for-people-whose-plans-have-been-canceled/.

[5] Ken Terry, "Health Insurance Exchanges Plagued By Data Errors," Information Week, October 11, 2013, available at http://www.informationweek.com/healthcare/electronic-health-records/health-insurance-exchanges-plagued-by-data-errors/d/d-id/1111910?; Irving Dejohn, "Fort Collins man accidentally signs up dog for health care," *New York Daily News*, November 2013, available at http://www.nydailynews.com/news/national/colorado-dog-accidentally-health-care-article-1.1523268; David Martosko, "'They had no idea if my insurance was active or not!': ObamaCare confusion reigns as frustrated patients walk out of hospitals without treatment," *Daily Mail* online, January 3, 2014, available at http://www.dailymail.co.uk/news/article-2532869/They-no-idea-insurance-active-not-At-Virginia-hospitals-ObamaCare-confusion-reigns-frustrated-patients-walk-out.html; and Sarah Kliff, "HealthCare.gov finally works — for some people," *Washington Post*, Wonkblog, December 2, 2013, available at http://www.washingtonpost.com/blogs/wonkblog/wp/2013/12/02/healthcare-gov-finally-works-for-some-people/.

[6] Kyle Blaine, "Sen. Rand Paul Says ObamaCare 'A Mess,' Unsure if Family is Covered," ABC News, January 5, 2014. Available at http://abcnews.go.com/blogs/politics/2014/01/sen-rand-paul-says-ObamaCare-a-mess-unsure-if-family-is-covered/.

[7] Ricardo Alonso-Zaldivar, "Adding baby to ObamaCare health plan isn't easy," Associated Press, January 3, 2014. Available at http://www.nbcnews.com/health/adding-baby-ObamaCare-health-plan-isnt-easy-2D11848994.

8   Sarah Kliff, "These Two Paragraphs Say Everything about Healthcare. Gov's Problems," *Washington Post*, December 3, 2013. Available at http://www.washingtonpost.com/blogs/wonkblog/wp/2013/12/03/these-two-paragraphs-say-everything-about-healthcare-govs-problems-2/.

9   David Martosko, "'They had no idea if my insurance was active or not!': ObamaCare confusion reigns as frustrated patients walk out of hospitals without treatment," *Daily Mail* online, January 2, 2014, available at http://www.dailymail.co.uk/news/article-2532869/They-no-idea-insurance-active-not-At-Virginia-hospitals-ObamaCare-confusion-reigns-frustrated-patients-walk-out.html; and Sarah Kliff and Sandhya Somashekhar, "Health Insurance Marketplaces Will Not Be Required to Verify Consumer Claims," *Washington Post*, July 5, 2013, available at http://www.washingtonpost.com/national/health-science/health-insurance-marketplaces-will-not-be-required-to-verify-consumer-claims/2013/07/05/d2a171f4-e5ab-11e2-aef3-339619eab080_story.html.

10 Timothy W. Martin and Christopher Weaver, "Health insurers Race to complete Enrollment," *Wall Street Journal*, December 30, 2013. Available at http://online.wsj.com/news/articles/SB10001424052702304361604579290942095319848?mod=rss_US_News.

11 Shannon Firth, "AHIP Postpones ObamaCare Premium Deadline," U.S.News.com, December 18, 2013. Available at http://www.usnews.com/news/articles/2013/12/18/ahip-postpones-ObamaCare-premium-deadline.

12 Patrick Morrisey, "How ObamaCare Makes Theft of Your Identity More Likely," *Forbes*, August 25, 2013. Available at http://www.forbes.com/sites/realspin/2013/08/25/how-ObamaCare-makes-theft-of-your-identity-more-likely/.

13 Larry Bell, "ACA Website Security Worries? Trust Us; We're with the Government," *Forbes*, December 29, 2013. Available at http://www.forbes.com/sites/larrybell/2013/12/29/aca-website-security-worries-trust-us-were-with-the-government/.

14 Adam Brandon, "Brandon: A gift from the federal shutdown," *Washington Post*, December 25, 2013, available at http://www.washingtontimes.com/news/2013/dec/25/brandon-a-gift-from-the-federal-shutdown/; see also Jason Millman, "Kathleen Sebelius pushes back against GOP critics," Politico.com, December 11, 2013, available at http://www.politico.com/story/2013/12/sebelius-ObamaCare-website-investigation-100999.html.

15 Robert Laszewski, "Healthcare.Gov's Numbers at the Deadline," Healthcare Blog, December 30, 2013. Available at http://thehealthcareblog.com/blog/2013/12/30/healthcare-govs-numbers-at-the-deadline/.

[16] Edie Littlefield Sundby, "You Also Can't Keep Your Doctor," *Wall Street Journal*, November 3, 2013. Available at http://online.wsj.com/news/articles/SB10001424052702304527504579171710423780446.

[17] John C. Goodman, "ObamaCares Insurance Exchanges Will Foster a Race to the Healthcare Bottom," *Forbes*, September 25, 2013. Available at http://www.ncpa.org/commentaries/ObamaCare-s-insurance-exchanges-will-foster-a-race-to-the-healthcare-bottom.

[18] "CBO's May 2013 Estimate of the Effects of the Affordable Care Act on Health Insurance Coverage," Congressional Budget Office, May, 2013, Table 1. Available at http://www.cbo.gov/sites/default/files/cbofiles/attachments/44190_EffectsAffordableCareActHealthInsuranceCoverage_2.pdf.

[19] Robert E. Moffit, Ph.D. and Alyene Senger, "The Obama Medicare Agenda: Why Seniors Will Fare Worse," Heritage Foundation, Backgrounder #2801, May 23, 2013; Douglas W. Elmendorf, CBO Letter to Speaker John Boehner, July 24, 2012. Available http://www.cbo.gov/sites/default/files/cbofiles/attachments/43471-hr6079.pdf.

[20] Richard S. Foster, "Estimated Financial Effects of the 'Patient Protection and Affordable Care Act,' as Amended," Centers for Medicare and Medicaid Services, April 22, 2010. Available at http://republicans.waysandmeans.house.gov/UploadedFiles/ Oact_Memorandum_on_Financial_Impact_of_PPact_as_Enacted.pdf.

[21] "Five Unaffordable Facts About the New Health Care Law: the Patient Protection and Affordable Care Act," National Federation of Independent Business, April 2010. Available at http://health.burgess.house.gov/uploadedfiles/nfib_-_5_unaffordable_facts_about_health_reform_law.pdf.

[22] John C. Goodman, "The Senate Health Bill," John Goodman's Health Policy Blog, December 9, 2009. Available at http://www.john-goodman-blog.com/the-senate-health-bill/.

[23] Douglas Elmendorf, "Testimony before the House Budget Committee," February 12, 2011, available at http://www.youtube.com/watch?v=QlBvrp4qV7Q&feature=player_embedded; and Chris Conover, "Healthcare Law Will Cost 1 Million or More Jobs," Forbes Pharma & Healthcare Blog, July 31, 2012, available at http://www.forbes.com/sites/chrisconover/2012/07/31/healthcare-law-will-cost-1-million-or-more-jobs/.

[24] Douglas Elmendorf, "Health Costs and the Federal Budget," Congressional Budget Office Director's Blog, May 28, 2010. Available at http://cboblog.cbo.gov/?p=1034.

[25] Andrea M. Sisko et al., "National Health Spending Projections: The Estimated Impact Of Reform Through 2019," *Health Affairs*, Vol. 29, September 2010. Available at http://content.healthaffairs.org/content/29/9/1714.abstract.

26 Jeanne S. Ringel et al., "Analysis of the Patient Protection and Affordable Care Act (H.R. 3590)," Policy Brief, RAND Corporation, 2010. Available at http://www.rand.org/pubs/research_briefs/2010/RAND_RB9514.pdf.

27 Jonathan Gruber, "When will we get the verdict on ObamaCare?" CNN. com, January 2, 2014. Available at http://www.cnn.com/2014/01/02/opinion/gruber-aca-success/.

28 Joseph Antos, "Containing health care costs: Recent progress and remaining challenges," testimony before the Senate, July 30, 2013. Available at http://www.aei.org/speech/health/healthcare-reform/containing-health-care-costs-recent-progress-and-remaining-challenges/?utm_source=Scholar&utm_medium=Paramount&utm_campaign=containing-health-care-costs.

29 John D. Shatto and M. Kent Clemens, "Projected Medicare Expenditures under an Illustrative Scenario with Alternative Payment Updates to Medicare Providers," Centers for Medicare & Medicaid Services, August 5, 2010. Available at http://www.cms.gov/ReportsTrustFunds/downloads/2010TRAlternativeScenario.pdf.

30 Joseph P. Newhouse, "Assessing Health Reform's Impact on Four Key Groups of Americans," *Health Affairs*, Vol. 29, No. 9, September 10, 2010. Available at http://content.healthaffairs.org/cgi/content/abstract/hlthaff.2010.0595.

31 Ibid. Also see Jim Hahn, "Medicare Physician Payment Updates and the Sustainable Growth Rate (SGR) System Analyst in Health Care Financing," Congressional Research Service, April 9, 2010. Available at http://op.bna.com/hl.nsf/id/droy-84frgj/$File/CRS%20report%20sustainable%20growth%20rate.pdf.

32 John C. Goodman, "Health Savings Accounts Will Revolutionize American Health Care," National Center for Policy Analysis, Brief Analysis No. 464, January 15, 2004. Available at http://www.ncpa.org/pdfs/ba464.pdf.

33 Devon M. Herrick, "ObamaCare Penalty May Contribute To Decline Of Marriage," *Investor's Business Daily*, November 11, 06, 2013. Available at http://news.investors.com/ibd-editorials-perspective/110613-678212-hidden-in-ObamaCare-is-penalty-against-marriage.htm.

34 Devon M. Herrick, "Health Exchange Subsidies Will Reduce Employer Health Plans," National Center for Policy Analysis, Brief Analysis No. 758, November 16, 2011. Available at http://www.ncpa.org/pdfs/st134.pdf.

35 Jack Hadley and John Holahan, "Covering the Uninsured: How Much Would it Cost?" *Health Affairs*, Web Exclusive, June 4, 2003, pages W325-265. Available at http://content.healthaffairs.org/cgi/content/abstract/hlthaff.w3.250v1.

36 "CBO's May 2013 Estimate of the Effects of the Affordable Care Act on Health Insurance Coverage," Congressional Budget Office, May, 2013,

Table 1. Available at http://www.cbo.gov/sites/default/files/cbofiles/ attachments/44190_EffectsAffordableCareActHealthInsuranceCoverage_ 2.pdf.

[37] Richard S. Foster, "Estimated Financial Effects of the 'Patient Protection and Affordable Care Act,' as Amended." And Carla K. Johnson, "Health Overhaul May Mean Longer ER Waits, Crowding," *USA Today*, July 2, 2010 available at http://www.usatoday.com/news/health/2010-07-02-emergency-room_N.htm.

[38] Catherine Arnst, "A New Practice: The Doctor Will See You Today," *Boston Globe*, July 14, 2010. Available at http://www.boston.com/ yourtown/cambridge/articles/2010/07/14/a_new_practice_the_doctor_ will_see_you_today/. See also "2009 Survey of Physician Appointment Wait Times," Merritt Hawkins & Associates, May 2009. Available at http://www.merritthawkins.com/pdf/mha2009waittimesurvey.pdf.

[39] "Hospital Inpatient and Emergency Utilization Trends FY04-FY08," Publication No. 10-352-HCF-01, Division of Health Care Finance and Policy, Commonwealth of Massachusetts, June 2010. Available at http:// www.mass.gov/Eeohhs2/docs/dhcfp/r/pubs/10/hospital_inpatient%20 and_ed_%20util_06-30-10.doc.

[40] Katherine Baicker and the Oregon Health Study Group, "The Oregon Experiment — Effects of Medicaid on Clinical Outcomes," *New England Journal of Medicine*, Vol. 386, No. 18, May 2, 2013. Available at http:// www.nejm.org/doi/full/10.1056/NEJMsa1212321.

[41] Christian S. Spencer, Darrell J. Gaskin and Eric T. Roberts, "The Quality of Care Delivered to Patients Within The Same Hospital Varies By Insurance Type," *Health Affairs*, October 2013. Available at http:// content.healthaffairs.org/content/32/10/1731.abstract.

[42] Jack Hadley et al., "Medical Spending and the Health of the Elderly," Wiley Online Library, Health Services Research Vol. 46, Issue 5, Pages 1333-1361, May 24, 2011. Available at http://onlinelibrary.wiley.com/ doi/10.1111/j.1475-6773.2011.01276.x/abstract.

[43] Vivian Y. Wu, Yu-Chu Shen, "The Long-term Impact of Medicare Payment Reductions on Patient Outcomes," National Bureau of Economic Research, Working Paper No. 16859, March 2011. Available at http://www.NBER.org/papers/w16859.

[44] John C. Goodman, "Will the Affordable Care Act Cause Seniors to Die Early?," John Goodman's Health Policy Blog, June 6, 2011. Available at http://healthblog.ncpa.org/the-affordable-care-act-causes-seniors-to-die/.

[45] John C. Goodman, "Why the Pilot Programs Failed," John Goodman's Health Policy Blog, January 30, 2012, available at http://healthblog.ncpa. org/why-the-pilot-programs-failed/; John C. Goodman, "CBO: Obama Care Reforms Will Not Control Costs," John Goodman's Health Policy Blog, July 14, 2011, available at http://healthblog.ncpa.org/cbo-obama-care-reforms-

will-not-control-costs/; and John C. Goodman, "CBO: Pilot Programs Aren't Working," John Goodman's Health Policy Blog, January 19, 2012, available at http://healthblog.ncpa.org/cbo-pilot-programs-arent-working/.

46 Robert Pear, "Lower Health Insurance Premiums to Come at Cost of Fewer Choices," *New York Times*, September 22, 2013. Available at http://www.nytimes.com/2013/09/23/health/lower-health-insurance-premiums-to-come-at-cost-of-fewer-choices.html.

47 Sarah L. Taubman et al., "Medicaid Increases Emergency-Department Use: Evidence from Oregon's Health Insurance Experiment," *Advancing Science, Serving Society*, January 2, 2014; available at http://www.sciencemag.org/content/early/2014/01/02/science.1246183.

48 Sabrina Tavernise, "Cuts in Hospital Subsidies Threaten Safety-Net Care," *New York Times*, November 8, 2013; available at http://www.nytimes.com/2013/11/09/health/cuts-in-hospital-subsidies-threaten-safety-net-care.html?pagewanted=1&_r=0.

49 David C. Dugdale, Ronald Epstein and Steven Z. Pantilat, "Time and the Patient-Physician Relationship," *Journal of General Internal Medicine*, Society of General Internal Medicine, Vol. 14, No. S1, January 1999, pages S34-S40. Available at http://ukpmc.ac.uk/articles/PMC1496869;jsessionid=3777EB9730209893C721767CBDB69BC4.jvm4.

50 Centers for Medicare & Medicaid Services "What are my preventive care benefits: Part 1?," Healthcare.gov, 2014. Available at https://www.healthcare.gov/what-are-my-preventive-care-benefits/.

51 Louise B. Russell, "Preventing Chronic Disease: An Important Investment, But Don't Count On Cost Savings," *Health Affairs*, Vol. 28, No. 1, January / February 2009, pages 42-45. Available at http://content.healthaffairs.org/cgi/content/abstract/28/1/42. See also John C. Goodman, Gerald L. Musgrave and Devon M. Herrick, *Lives at Risk: Single-Payer National Health Insurance Around the World* (Lanham, Md.: Rowman & Littlefield, 2004), Chapter 12. Available at http://www.ncpa.org/pdfs/livesatrisk/ch12.pdf.

52 Libby Purves, "NHS Rationing is a Reality We Should Deal With," *Times (UK)*, August 11, 2008. Available at http://www.timesonline.co.uk/tol/comment/columnists/libby_purves/article4498748.ece.

53 Robert Laszewski, "Healthcare.Gov's Numbers at the Deadline."

54 "Amendment to Regulation on 'Grandfathered' Health Plans under the Affordable Care Act," U.S. Department of Health and Human Services. Available at http://www.hhs.gov/cciio/regulations/grandfather/factsheet.html.

55 Charles C. Johnson, "Obama admin repeatedly modified 'grandfathering' rules to benefit big business, not individuals," *Daily Caller*, November 4, 2013. Available at http://dailycaller.com/2013/11/04/obama-admin-repeatedly-modified-grandfathering-rules-to-benefit-big-business-not-individuals/.

56 HealthReform.Gov, "Fact Sheet: Keeping the Health Plan You Have: The Affordable Care Act and 'Grandfathered' Health Plans," U.S. Department of Health and Human Services, August 2, 2010. Available at http://www.healthreform.gov/newsroom/keeping_the_health_plan_you_have.html.

57 Hewitt Associates, "Nine out of 10 U.S. Companies Anticipate Losing Grandfather Status Under Health Care Reform, According to New Hewitt Survey," Press Release, August 2010. Available at http://www.hewittassociates.com/Intl/NA/en-US/AboutHewitt/Newsroom/PressReleaseDetail.aspx?cid=8810.

58 Paul Keckley et al., "2012 Deloitte Survey of U.S. Employers: Opinions about the U.S. Health Care System and Plans for Employee Health Benefits," Deloitte Center for Health Solutions, Deloitte Consulting, July 2012. Available at http://www.deloitte.com/assets/Dcom-UnitedStates/Local%20Assets/Documents/us_dchs_employee_survey_072512.pdf.

59 Louise Radnofsky, "Deloitte: One in 10 U.S. Employers to Drop Health Coverage, *Wall Street Journal*, July 24, 2012. Available at http://online.wsj.com/article/SB10000872396390443437504577545770682810842.html.

60 Jessica Banthin, Holly Harvey and Jean Hearne, "Estimates for the Insurance Coverage Provisions of the Affordable Care Act Updated for the Recent Supreme Court Decision," Congressional Budget Office, July 24, 2012. Available at http://www.cbo.gov/sites/default/files/cbofiles/attachments/43472-07-24-2012-CoverageEstimates.pdf.

61 Richard S. Foster, "Estimated Financial Effects of the 'Patient Protection and Affordable Care Act,' as Amended."

62 Douglas Holtz-Eakin and Cameron Smith, "Labor Markets and Health Care Reform: New Results," American Action Forum, May 2010. Available at http://americanactionforum.org/sites/default/files/OHC_LabMktsHCR.pdf.

63 Richard S. Foster, "Estimated Financial Effects of the 'Patient Protection and Affordable Care Act,' as Amended."

64 Sam Baker, "HHS Finalizes Over 1,200 Waivers Under Healthcare Reform Law," *The Hill*, January 06, 2012. Available at http://thehill.com/blogs/healthwatch/health-reform-implementation/202791-hhs-finalizes-more-than-1200-healthcare-waivers.

65 "What the Actuarial Values in the Affordable Care Act Mean," Kaiser Family Foundation, April 1, 2011. Available at http://kaiserfamilyfoundation.files.wordpress.com/2013/01/8177.pdf.

66 Richard Pollock, "Doctors boycotting California's ObamaCare exchange," *Washington Examiner*, December 6, 2013. Available at http://washingtonexaminer.com/doctors-boycotting-californias-ObamaCare-exchange/article/2540272.

[67] Barry P. Simmons et al., "The Massachusetts health care reform experience: What you need to know," *Orthopedics Today*, April 2010. Availableathttp://www.healio.com/orthopedics/business-of-orthopedics/news/print/orthopedics-today/%7Bd1f70aa0-d803-4227-857d-12a076540b44%7D/the-massachusetts-health-care-reform-experience-what-you-need-to-know.

[68] Jed Graham, "ObamaCare Has Separate Risk Pool For Young Adults," *Investor's Business Daily*, November 20, 2013. Available at http://news.investors.com/politics-ObamaCare/112013-680080-ObamaCare-catastrophic-risk-pools-fuels-adverse-selection.htm.

[69] Amy Goldstein, "Obama administration relaxes rules of health-care law four days before deadline," *Washington Post*, December 19, 2013. http://www.washingtonpost.com/national/health-science/obama-administration-relaxes-rules-of-health-care-law-four-days-before-deadline/2013/12/19/81bc3132-690b-11e3-8b5b-a77187b716a3_story.html.

[70] Douglas W. Elmendorf and Philip Ellis, "Estimated Premiums for "Bronze" Coverage Under the Patient Protection and Affordable Care Act," Congressional Budget Office, Letter to Honorable Olympia Snowe, January 11, 2010. Available at http://www.cbo.gov/sites/default/files/cbofiles/ftpdocs/108xx/doc10884/01-11-premiums_for_bronze_plan.pdf.

[71] Douglas W. Elmendorf, CBO Letter to Chairman Charles B. Rangel, November 2, 2009. Available at http://energycommerce.house.gov/Press_111/health_care/hr3962_CBOLetter.pdf.

[72] "'Average' Exchange Premiums Come In Lower Than Projected," *Kaiser Health News*, September 25, 2013. Available http://www.kaiserhealthnews.org/Daily-Reports/2013/September/25/premium-estimates-lower-than-expected.aspx.

[73] Steve Davis, "Exchanges May Face Backlash Over Subsidy Overpayment 'Clawback,'" *Health Business Daily*, Vol. 1, Issue 1, August 2011. Available at http://aishealth.com/archive/nhex0811-06.

[74] Ibid.

[75] Katie Thomas, Reed Abelson and Jo Craven McGinty, "New Health Law Frustrates Many in Middle Class," *New York Times*, December 20, 2013. Available at http://www.nytimes.com/2013/12/21/business/new-health-law-frustrates-many-in-middle-class.html.

[76] Ibid. See also Sam Baker, "Issa probes talks between White House, IRS on healthcare law," *The Hill*, August 22, 2012. Available at http://thehill.com/blogs/healthwatch/health-reform-implementation/244825-issa-probes-talks-between-white-house-irs-on-healthcare-law.

[77] Stephen Miller, "Final Rule Provides Wellness Incentive Guidance," Society for Human Resource Management, June 5, 2013. Available at http://www.shrm.org/hrdisciplines/benefits/articles/pages/final-rule-wellness-programs.aspx.

[78] Timothy Jost, "Implementing Health Reform: Allowing Consumers With Nonrenewed Policies To Buy Catastrophic Coverage And Other Developments," *Health Affairs*, December 20, 2013. Available at http://healthaffairs.org/blog/2013/12/20/implementing-health-reform-allowing-consumers-with-nonrenewed-policies-to-buy-catastrophic-coverage-and-other-developments/.

[79] Sarah Kliff and Ezra Klein, "Everything you need to know about life under ObamaCare," *Washington Post*, Wonkblog, January 1, 2014. Available at http://www.washingtonpost.com/blogs/wonkblog/wp/2014/01/01/everything-you-need-to-know-about-life-under-ObamaCare-2/.

[80] Matt Nesto, "Beware of ObamaCare? IBM Joins Growing List of Employers Giving Cause for Concern," Yahoo Finance, September 9, 2013. Available at http://finance.yahoo.com/blogs/breakout/ibm-joins-growing-list-employers-booting-retirees-health-160604063.html.

[81] Alex Nussbaum, "GE, IBM Ending Retiree Health Plans in Historic Shift," Bloomberg.com, September 9, 2013. Available at http://www.bloomberg.com/news/2013-09-09/ge-to-ibm-ending-retiree-health-plans-in-historic-shift.html.

[82] Brigitte Madrian, "Employment-Based Health Insurance and Job Mobility: Is There Evidence of Job-Lock?," *Quarterly Journal of Economics*, Vol. 109, No. 1, 1994, pages 27-54; Jonathan Gruber and Brigitte Madrian "Health Insurance, Labor Supply, and Job Mobility: A Critical Review," in Catherine McLaughlin, ed., *Health Policy and the Uninsured* (Washington, D.C.: Urban University Press, 2004), pages 97-178.

[83] Steven Greenhouse and Jonathan Martin, "Unions' Misgivings on Health Law Burst Into View," *New York Times*, September 11, 2013. Available athttp://www.nytimes.com/2013/09/12/business/unions-misgivings-on-health-law-burst-into-view.html.

[84] Doug Badger, "More Than A Website: Will Insurers Prosper Under ObamaCare?" Brief Case blog, October 28, 2013. Available at http://www.dougsbriefcase.com/blog/website-will-insurers-prosper-ObamaCare/.

[85] Elise Viebeck, "Unions might dodge ObamaCare tax," *The Hill*, November 06, 2013. http://thehill.com/blogs/healthwatch/health-reform-implementation/189413-labor-unions-may-get-tax-wish-on-ObamaCare. Also see John C. Goodman, "'The Belly Button Tax," John Goodman's Health Policy Blog, November 1, 2013. Available at http://www.dougsbriefcase.com/blog/website-will-insurers-prosper-ObamaCare/http://healthblog.ncpa.org/the-belly-button-tax/.

[86] Ezra Klein, "Obama administration denies labor's request for health care waiver," *Washington Post*, Wonkblog, September 13. Available at

http://www.washingtonpost.com/blogs/wonkblog/wp/2013/09/13/obama-administration-denies-labors-request-for-health-care-waiver/.

87 Gina Kolata, "Co-Payments Soar for Drugs with High Prices," *New York Times*, April 14, 2008. Available at http://www.nytimes.com/2008/04/14/us/14drug.html.

88 John C. Goodman, "Why the Exchanges are a Mess and a Very Simple Solution," John Goodman's Health Policy Blog, October 28, 2013. Available at http://healthblog.ncpa.org/why-the-exchanges-are-a-mess-and-a-very-simple-solution/.

89 "State Actions to Address Health Insurance Exchanges," National Conference of State Legislatures, December 30, 2013. http://www.ncsl.org/research/health/state-actions-to-implement-the-health-benefit.aspx.

90 John C. Goodman, "Navigating the ObamaCare Maze," *Wall Street Journal*, May 20, 2013. Available at http://www.ncpa.org/pdfs/20130520_Navigating_the_ObamaCare_Maze-WSJ-op-ed.pdf.

91 Hannah Winston, "Veterans Affairs, Defense Depts. spend billions in effort to coordinate records," Center for Public Integrity, August 27, 2013. Available at http://www.publicintegrity.org/2013/08/27/13253/veterans-affairs-defense-depts-spend-billions-effort-coordinate-records.

92 Patricia Kime, "VA, DoD pull back on electronic health records," *Army Times*, February 6, 2013. Available at http://www.armytimes.com/article/20130206/BENEFITS04/302060312/VA-DoD-pull-back-on-electronic-health-records.

93 Chris Frates, "3 states tell insurers to scrap plans that don't comply with ObamaCare," CNN.com, October 30, 2013. Available at http://www.cnn.com/2013/10/29/politics/ObamaCare-states-scrap-insurance-plans/.

94 Gary Cohen, letter to state insurance commissioners, U.S. Department of Health and Human Services, November 14, 2013. Available at http://www.cms.gov/CCIIO/Resources/Letters/Downloads/commissioner-letter-11-14-2013.PDF.

95 John W. Schoen, "Want to keep your health plan? In most states, you can," NBC News, December 4, 2013. Available at http://www.nbcnews.com/health/want-keep-your-health-plan-most-states-you-can-2D11691633.

96 "Options Available for Consumers with Canceled Policies," U.S. Department of Health and Human Services, December 19, 2013. Available at http://www.cms.gov/CCIIO/Resources/Regulations-and-Guidance/Downloads/cancellation-consumer-options-12-19-2013.pdf.

97 Richard V. Burkhauser, Sean Lyons and Kosali I. Simon, "The Importance of the Meaning and Measurement of "Affordable" in the Affordable Care Act," National Bureau of Economic Research, Working Paper No. 17279, August 2011. Available at http://www..org/papers/w17279.

98 "Ways and Means Republicans' Report: Democrats' Health Care Bill Contains Massive Expansion of IRS's Power," Ways and Means Republicans, March 18, 2010. Available at http://republicans.waysandmeans.house.gov/News/DocumentSingle.aspx?DocumentID=176997.

99 "Internal Revenue Service, FY 2014 President's Budget," Available at http://www.treasury.gov/about/budget-performance/CJ14/10.%20IRS%20CJ%20FINAL%20v2.pdf.

100 Paul Starr, "The Mandate Miscalculation: Obama's health care blunder—and how to fix it," *New Republic*, December 14, 2011, available at http://www.tnr.com/article/politics/magazine/98554/individual-mandate-affordable-care-act; and Casey B. Mulligan, "The Power of the Individual Mandate," *New York Times*, Economix blog, October 23, 2013, available at http://economix.blogs.nytimes.com/2013/10/23/the-power-of-the-individual-mandate/. See also Senator Tom Coburn's (R-OK) discussion, "IRS Enforcement of Individual Mandate Destined for Failure?" available at http://www.coburn.senate.gov/public/index.cfm?a=Files.Serve&File_id=fd932516-3dc2-486f-a4de-81687c7c6915.

101 Mike Patton, "ObamaCare: Penalties And Exemptions," *Forbes* online, October 28, 2013. Available at http://www.forbes.com/sites/mikepatton/2013/10/28/ObamaCare-penalties-and-exemptions/. See also Jessica Banthin, Alexandra Minicozzi, Holly Harvey and Sarah Anders, "Payments of Penalties for Being Uninsured Under the Affordable Care Act," Congressional Budget Office, September 2012, available at http://www.cbo.gov/sites/default/files/cbofiles/attachments/Indiv_Mandate_Penalty_One-Col.pdf; and Timothy Jost, "Implementing Health Reform: Shared Responsibility Tax Exemptions and Family Coverage Affordability," *Health Affairs* blog, January 31, 2013, available at http://healthaffairs.org/blog/2013/01/31/implementing-health-reform-shared-responsibility-tax-exemptions-and-family-coverage-affordability/.

102 Aaron Carroll, "Lucky Duckies Who Are Exempt from the Individual Mandate," *Incidental Economist*, July 2, 2013. Available at http://theincidentaleconomist.com/wordpress/lucky-duckies-who-are-exempt-from-the-individual-mandate/.

103 Darius Tahir, "Narrow-Network Health Plans Expected to Proliferate Under ObamaCare."

104 Richard Pollock, "Doctors boycotting California's ObamaCare exchange."

105 James C. Robinson and Timothy T. Brown, "Increases in Consumer Cost Sharing Redirect Patient Volumes And Reduce Hospital Prices For Orthopedic Surgery," *Health Affairs*, Vol. 32, No. 8, August 2013, pages 1,392-97. Available at http://content.healthaffairs.org/content/32/8/1392.full.pdf+html.

[106] "CBO's May 2013 Estimate of the Effects of the Affordable Care Act on Health Insurance Coverage," Congressional Budget Office, May, 2013, Table 1. Available at http://www.cbo.gov/sites/default/files/cbofiles/attachments/44190_EffectsAffordableCareActHealthInsuranceCoverage_2.pdf.

[107] Jack Hadley and John Holahan, "Covering the Uninsured: How Much Would it Cost?"

[108] Tom Coburn and John Barrasso, "Bad Medicine: a Check-Up on the New Federal Health Law," July 2010. Available at http://coburn.senate.gov/public/index.cfm?a=Files.Serve&File_id=722faf8b-a5be-40fd-a52b-9a98826c1592.

[109] "HealthCare.gov," U.S. Department of Health and Human Services, 2010. Available at http://www.healthcare.gov/.

[110] Doug Trapp, "Primary Care Gets Boost with $250 Million in HHS Grants," *American Medical News*, July 1, 2010. Available at http://www.ama-assn.org/amednews/2010/06/28/gvsf0701.htm.

[111] Julian Pecquet, "Investment in Healthcare Workforce Announced as Doctor Shortage Looms," Healthwatch: the Hill's Healthcare Blog, June 16, 2010. Available at http://thehill.com/blogs/healthwatch/health-reform-implementation/103575-investment-in-healthcare-workforce-announced-as-doctor-shortage-looms.

[112] "Texas Nursing: Our Future Depends on It, A Strategic Plan for the State of Texas to Meet Nursing Workforce Needs of 2013," Texas Department of Health and Human Services, April 2010. Available at http://www.dshs.state.tx.us/chs/cnws/TexasTeam/TexasStrategy.pdf.

[113] Stephen Zuckerman, Aimee F. Williams and Karen E. Stockley, "Trends In Medicaid Physician Fees, 2003–2008," *Health Affairs*, Vol. 28, No. 3, April 28, 2009, pages W510-W519. Available at http://content.healthaffairs.org/cgi/content/abstract/ hlthaff.28.3.w510.

[114] John C. Goodman, "Emergency Room Visits Likely to Increase Under ObamaCare," National Center for Policy Analysis, Brief Analysis No. 709, June 18, 2010, available at http://www.ncpa.org/pdfs/ba709.pdf; and Michael Anderson, Carlos Dobkin and Tal Gross, "The Effect of Health Insurance Coverage on the Use of Medical Services," National Bureau of Economic Research, Working Paper No. 15823, March 2010. Available at http://www..org/papers/w15823.

[115] Tamyra Carroll Garcia, Amy B. Bernstein, and Mary Ann Bush, "Emergency Department Visitors and Visits: Who Used the Emergency Room in 2007?" National Center for Health Statistics, U.S. Centers for Disease Control and Prevention, Data Brief No. 38, May 2010. Available at http://www.cdc.gov/nchs/data/databriefs/db38.pdf.

[116] Scott Gottlieb, "The Doctor Won't See You Now. He's Clocked Out," *Wall Street Journal*, March 14, 2013. Available at http://online.wsj.com/article/SB10001424127887323628804578346614033833092.html.

[117] Anna Wilde Mathews, "Same Doctor Visit, Double the Cost," *Wall Street Journal*, August 27, 2012. Available at http://online.wsj.com/article/SB10 0008723963904437137045776011 13671007448.html.

[118] Atul Gawande, "The Velluvial Matrix," *New Yorker*, June 16, 2010. Availableathttp://www.newyorker.com/online/blogs/newsdesk/2010/06/gawande-stanford-speech.html.

[119] Karen Davis, "How Will the Health Care System Change Under Health Reform?" Commonwealth Fund Blog, June 29, 2010. Available at http://www.commonwealthfund.org/Content/Blog/How-Will-the-Health-Care-System-Change.aspx.

[120] Darius Tahir, "Narrow-Network Health Plans Expected to Proliferate Under ObamaCare," *National Journal*, October 9, 2013. Available at http://www.nationaljournal.com/innovations-in-health/narrow-network-health-plans-expected-to-proliferate-under-ObamaCare-20131009.

[121] Reed Abelson, "Insurers Push Plans That Limit Choice of Doctor," *New York Times*, July 17, 2010. Available at http://www.nytimes.com/2010/07/18/business/18choice.html.

[122] Uwe E. Reinhardt, Peter S. Hussey and Gerard F. Anderson, "U.S. Health Care Spending in an International Context: Why is U.S. spending so high, and can we afford it?" *Health Affairs*, Vol. 23, No. 3, May/June 2004, pages 10-25. Available at http://content.healthaffairs.org/cgi/reprint/23/3/10.

[123] "Preventive Services Covered under the Affordable Care Act," U.S. Department of Health and Human Services. Available at http://www.hhs.gov/healthcare/facts/factsheets/2010/07/preventive-services-list.html.

[124] Sara Rosenbaum, Emily Jones, Peter Shin and Leighton Ku, "National Health Reform: How Will Medically Underserved Communities Fare?" George Washington University School of Public Health and Health Services and RCHN Community Health Foundation Research Collaborative, Policy Research Brief No. 10, July 9, 2009. Available at http://sphhs.gwu.edu/departments/healthpolicy/DHP_Publications/pub_uploads/dhpPublication_5046C2DE-5056-9D20-3D2A570F2CF3F8B0.pdf.

[125] Kimberly S. H. Yarnall et al., "Primary Care: Is there Enough Time for Prevention?" *American Journal of Public Health*, Vol. 93, No. 4, April 2003. Available at http://www.ncbi.nlm.nih.gov/pmc/articles/PMC1447803/pdf/0930635.pdf.

[126] David Brown, "In the Balance," *Washington Post*, April 8, 2008. Available at http://www.washingtonpost.com/wp-dyn/content/article/2008/04/04/AR2008040403803.html.

[127] John C. Goodman, "An Obituary," John Goodman's Health Policy Blog, January 30, 2009. Available at http://www.john-goodman-blog.com/an-

obituary/.

[128] Louise B. Russell, "Preventing Chronic Disease: An Important Investment, But Don't Count On Cost Savings."

[129] "Breast Cancer Screening Recommendations for Women at Higher Risk," Susan G. Komen for the Cure, July 9, 2010. Available at http://ww5. komen.org/BreastCancer/RecommendationsforWomenwithHigherRisk. html.

[130] John C. Goodman, "Health Savings Accounts Will Revolutionize American Health Care."

[131] Ethan Bronner, "A Flood of Suits Fights Coverage of Birth Control," *New York Times*, January 26, 2013. Available at http://www.nytimes. com/2013/01/27/health/religious-groups-and-employers-battle-contraception-mandate.html.

[132] "Women's Preventive Services Guidelines," U.S. Department of Health and Human Services. Available at http://www.hrsa.gov/ womensguidelines/.

[133] Ethan Bronner, "A Flood of Suits Fights Coverage of Birth Control."

[134] "Contraceptive Coverage in the Health Care Law: Frequently Asked Questions," National Women's Law Center, May 22, 2013. Available at http://www.nwlc.org/resource/contraceptive-coverage-health-care-law-frequently-asked-questions.

[135] Bill Mears, "Court delays ObamaCare contraception mandate for 2 nonprofits," *CNN*, December 31, 2013. Available at http://politicalticker. blogs.cnn.com/2013/12/31/u-s-supreme-court-temporarily-exempts-colorado-church-affiliated-group-from-healthcare-laws-contraception-mandate/.

[136] Ashley McGuire, "Why some Catholics think Obama is a master of deception," *CNN*, December 30, 2013; available at http://www.cnn. com/2013/12/30/opinion/catholics-ObamaCare-opinion/.

[137] Susan A. Cohen, "Insurance Coverage of Abortion: The Battle to Date and the Battle to Come," *Guttmacher Policy Review*, Vol. 13, Number 4, Fall 2010. Available at http://www.guttmacher.org/pubs/gpr/13/4/ gpr130402.html.

[138] "The Patient Protection and Affordable Care Act (Public Law 111-148)," Government Printing Office, 2010, available at http://goo.gl/ipNH3; and "Health Care and Education Reconciliation Act of 2010 (Public Law 111–152)," Government Printing Office, 2010, available at http://goo.gl/ AjQn2.

[139] "Abortion Provisions in the Patient and Protection and Affordable Care Act," Planned Parenthood; available at http://www.ppaction. org/site/DocServer/Fact_Sheet_-_Abortion_and_ACA.pdf and

Sara A. Emmert, "Health care reform upsets both sides of abortion issue," LegislativeGazette.com, April 2010. Available at http://www. legislativegazette.com/Articles-c-2010-04-05-66541.113122_Health_ care_reform_upsetsboth_ sides_ of_ abortion_issue.html.

[140] Dale Sanders, "Patient Safety and Electronic Health Records," *Health System CIO*, April 20, 2010. Available at http://healthsystemcio. com/2010/04/20/patient-safety-and-electronic-health-records/.

[141] Fred Schulte and Emma Schwartz, "FDA Considers Regulating Safety of Electronic Health Systems: Reports of Patient Harm Include Six Deaths in Two Years," Huffington Post Investigative Fund, February 23, 2010. Available at http://www.publicintegrity.org/2010/02/23/7047/fda-considers-regulating-safety-electronic-health-systems.

[142] Richard Hillestad et al., "Can Electronic Medical Record Systems Transform Health Care? Potential Health Benefits, Savings and Costs," *Health Affairs*, Vol. 24, No. 5, September/October 2005, pages 1,103–17. Available at http://content.healthaffairs.org/cgi/reprint/24/5/1103.

[143] Jan Walker et al., "The Value of Health Care Information Exchange and Interoperability," *Health Affairs*, January 19, 2005. Available at http:// content.healthaffairs.org/cgi/content/full/hlthaff.w5.10/DC1.

[144] "Evidence on the Costs and Benefits of Health Information Technology," Congressional Budget Office, May 2008. Available at http://www.cbo. gov/ftpdocs/91xx/doc9168/05-20-HealthIT.pdf.

[145] Devon M. Herrick, Linda Gorman and John C. Goodman, "Health Information Technology: Benefits and Problems," National Center for Policy Analysis, Policy Report No. 327, April 2010. Available at http:// www.ncpa.org/pdfs/st327.pdf.

[146] Linda Gorman, "British EMR Experiment Ends in Failure," John Goodman's Health Policy Blog, National Center for Policy Analysis, September 30, 2011. Available at http://healthblog.ncpa.org/british-emr-experiment-ends-in-failure/.

[147] Martin Beckford, "Dismantling NHS computer scheme could cost more money," Telegraph (UK), September 22, 2011. Available at http://www. telegraph.co.uk/news/politics/8782301/Dismantling-NHS-computer-scheme-could-cost-more-money.html.

[148] Pamela Lewis Dolan, "Laws bolster penalties for privacy breaches in California," *American Medical News*, December 1, 2008. Available at http://www.ama-assn.org/amednews/2008/12/01/bisa1201.htm.

[149] Charles Ornstein, "Fawcett's Cancer File Breached," *Los Angeles Times*, April 3, 2008. Available at http://articles.latimes.com/2008/apr/03/local/ me-farrah3.

[150] Richard O. Mason, "A Tapestry of Privacy: A Meta-Discussion," Privacy: Looking Ahead, Looking Back Connelly Program in Business Ethics, Georgetown School of Business. Available at http://cyberethics.cbi.

msstate.edu/mason2/.

[151] Mark Aitken, "Medical records of Gordon Brown and Alex Salmond hacked," *Daily Record* (UK), March 1, 2009. Available at http://www. dailyrecord.co.uk/news/scottish-news/2009/03/01/medical-records-of-gordon-brown-and-alex-salmond-hacked-78057-21162440/.

[152] Matthew J. Belvedere, "No security ever built into ObamaCare site: Hacker," CNBC.com, November 25, 2013 Available at http://www.cnbc. com/id/101225308.

[153] Walecia Konrad, "Medical Problems Could Include Identity Theft," *New York Times*, June 12, 2009. Available at http://www.nytimes. com/2009/06/13/health/13patient.html.

[154] Ibid.

[155] Eric Boehm, "feds not required to report security breaches of ObamaCare exchange website," *Foxnews*, December 5, 2013; available at http://www.foxnews.com/politics/2013/12/05/feds-not-required-to-report-security-breaches-ObamaCare-exchange-website/.

[156] Douglas W. Elmendorf, Letter to House Speaker Nancy Pelosi, Congressional Budget Office, March 20, 2010. Available at http://www. cbo.gov/ftpdocs/113xx/doc11379/AmendReconProp.pdf.

[157] Republican Finance Committee Staff calculations of the Joint Committee on Taxation Distributional Analysis of the Premium Credit, High Cost Plan Tax, Medical Expense Deduction, and the Medicare HI Tax, in the Patient Protection and Affordable Care Act. For a discussion with breakdown see Keith Hennessy, "How Would the Reid Bill Affect the Middle Class?" KeithHennessy.com, December 10, 2009. Available at http://keithhennessey.com/2009/12/10/reid-bill-middle-class/.

[158] Sam Brownback and Kevin Brady, "New Tax Could Boost Small Business Premiums an Extra $1,000 a Year," Joint Economic Committee, April 22, 2010. Available at http://jec.senate.gov/ republicans/public/?a=Files.Serve&File_id=1d63d12d-0e1b-45ee-8633-e3624a8ddcd4.

[159] "PPACA Implementation Timeline: What to Expect and When," National Federation of Independent Business, July 27, 2102. Available at http:// www.nfib.com/advocacy/item?cmsid=60471.

[160] CBO Letter to John Boehner, Speaker of the House of Representatives, Congressional Budget Office, July 24, 2012. Available at http://www.cbo. gov/sites/default/files/cbofiles/attachments/43471-hr6079.pdf.

[161] Ibid.

[162] Richard S. Foster, "Estimated Financial Effects of the 'Patient Protection and Affordable Care Act,' as Amended."

[163] Richard S. Foster, "Estimated Financial Effects of the 'Patient Protection and Affordable Care Act,' as passed by the Senate on December

24, 2009." Centers for Medicare and Medicaid Services, January 8, 2010. Available at http://www.politico.com/static/PPM130_oact_memorandum_on_senate_bill_as_passed_01-08-09.html.

164 Ricardo Alonso-Zaldivar, "More than 3M seniors may have to switch drug plans," Associated Press, August 25, 2010. Available at http://www.boston.com/business/healthcare/articles/2010/08/25/more_than_3m_seniors_may_have_to_switch_drug_plans/.

165 John C. Goodman, "ObamaCare Slams Employers, Retirees," John Goodman's Health Policy Blog, March 29, 2010. Available at http://www.john-goodman-blog.com/ObamaCare-slams-employers-retirees/.

166 "Comparison of Projected Medicare Part D Premiums Under Current Law and Under Reconciliation Legislation Combined with H.R. 3590 as Passed by the Senate," Congressional Budget Office, March 19, 2010. Available at http://www.cbo.gov/ftpdocs/113xx/doc11355/Comparison.pdf.

167 Jeffrey H. Anderson, "Sebelius Says GAO Report Is 'Just Not Accurate' — Then Helps Confirm That It Is," *Weekly Standard*, May 4, 2012. http://www.weeklystandard.com/keyword/Medicare-Advantage.

168 Sandhya Somashekhar, "U.S. to boost rather than cut payments to health insurers," *Washington Post*, April 1, 2013, http://www.washingtonpost.com/national/health-science/us-to-boost-rather-than-cut-payments-to-health-insurers/2013/04/01/7423c3a0-9b16-11e2-9a79-eb5280c81c63_story.html.

169 Thomas R. Saving, "How Will the Affordable Care Act Affect the Elderly and Disabled on Medicare?" PowerPoint presentation, NCPA Social Security Trustees Briefing, September 2010. Available at http://www.ncpa.org/pdfs/NCPA-Social-Security-Trustees-Briefing-2010.pdf.

170 John D. Shatto and M. Kent Clemens, "Projected Medicare Expenditures under an Illustrative Scenario with Alternative Payment Updates to Medicare Providers."

171 Todd Ackerman, "Texas doctors opting out of Medicare at alarming rate," *Houston Chronicle*, May 17, 2010. Available at http://www.chron.com/disp/story.mpl/metropolitan/7009807.html.

172 "Medicare and the Mayo Clinic: The famous hospital will no longer take some senior patients," *Wall Street Journal*, January 8, 2010. Available at http://online.wsj.com/article/SB100014240527487034365045746407116558861 36.html.

173 Joseph P. Newhouse, "Assessing Health Reform's Impact On Four Key Groups Of Americans."

174 Adam Atherly and Kenneth E. Thorpe, "The Impact of Reductions in Medicare Advantage Funding on Beneficiaries," Rollins School of Public Health, Emory University, April 2007. Available at http://c0540862.cdn.cloudfiles.rackspacecloud.com/Medicare_Advantage.pdf.

[175] Ibid. Also see Adam Atherly and Kenneth E. Thorpe, "Value of Medicare Advantage to Low-Income and Minority Beneficiaries," Rollins School of Public Health, Emory University, September 20, 2005.

[176] "Working Paper: A Preliminary Comparison of Utilization Measures Among Diabetes and Heart Disease Patients in Eight Regional Medicare Advantage Plans and Medicare Fee-for-Service in the Same Service Areas," AHIP Center for Policy and Research, September 2009. Available at http://www.ahipresearch.org/pdfs/MAvsFFS.pdf.

[177] Kathleen Sebelius, "Op-Ed: Securing Medicare's Future," Yahoo! News, July 29, 2010.

[178] Douglas W. Elmendorf, Letter to Senator Jeff Sessions, January 22, 2010. Available at http://www.cbo.gov/ftpdocs/110xx/ doc11005/01-22-HI_Fund.pdf.

[179] Richard S. Foster, "Estimated Financial Effects of the 'Patient Protection and Affordable Care Act,' as Amended."

[180] "Affordable Care Act Update: Implementing Medicare Cost Savings," Centers for Medicare & Medicaid Services, U.S. Department of Health and Human Services, August 2, 2010. Available at http://www.cms.gov/apps/docs/act-Update-Implementing-Medicare-Costs-Savings.pdf.

[181] "Mayberry Misleads on Medicare," FactCheck.org, the Annenberg Public Policy Center, July 31, 2010. Available at http://www.factcheck.org/2010/07/mayberry-misleads-on-medicare/.

[182] Chris Jacobs, "AARP's Health Care Bailouts," Republican Policy Committee, April 19, 2010. Available at http://www.ncpa.org/pdfs/E-mail-from-Chris-Jacobs-RPC.pdf.

[183] Devon M. Herrick, "Exchanging Medicaid for Private Insurance," National Center for Policy Analysis, Policy Report No. 343, December 14, 2012. Available at http://www.ncpa.org/pub/st343.

[184] "11.5 Million Poor Uninsured Americans Could Be Eligible for Medicaid if States Opt for ACA Expansion," Health Policy Center, Urban Institute, Fourth Quarter 2013. Available at http://www.urban.org/health_policy/health_care_reform/map.cfm.

[185] Brent R. Asplin et al., "Insurance Status and Access to Urgent Ambulatory Care Follow-up Appointments," *Journal of the American Medical Association*, Vol. 294, No. 10, September 14, 2005. Available at http://jama.ama-assn.org/cgi/content/abstract/294/10/1248.

[186] "2009 Survey of Physician Appointment Wait Times," Merritt Hawkins and Associates, 2009. Available at http://www.merritthawkins.com/pdf/mha2009waittimesurvey.pdf.

[187] Tamyra Carroll Garcia, Amy B. Bernstein and Mary Ann Bush, "Emergency Department Visitors and Visits: Who Used the Emergency Room in 2007?" Centers for Disease Control and Prevention, National

Center for Health Statistics, Data Brief No. 38, May 2010. Available at http://www.cdc.gov/nchs/data/databriefs/ db38. pdf.

[188] Avik Roy, "UVA Study: Surgical Patients on Medicaid Are 13% More Likely to Die Than Those Without Insurance," *National Review*, July 17, 2010. Available at http://www.nationalreview.com/critical-condition/231147/uva-study-surgical-patients-medicaid-are-13-more-likely-die-those-without-.

[189] Damien J. LaPar et al., "Primary Payer Status Affects Mortality for Major Surgical Operations," Presentation to the 130th Annual Meeting of the American Surgical Association, 130th Annual Meeting Abstracts, April 2010. Available at http://www.americansurgical.info/abstracts/2010/18.cgi.

[190] Richard G. Roetzheim et al., "Effects of Health Insurance and Race on Early Detection of Cancer," *Journal of the National Cancer Institute*, August 18, 1999. Available at http://jnci.oxfordjournals.org/cgi/content/full/91/16/1409?ijkey=3894238ad956b166ab570c56f9648d625979f6d4.

[191] Rachel Rapaport Kelz et al., "Morbidity and Mortality of Colorectal Carcinoma Surgery Differs by Insurance Status," *Cancer*, Vol. 101, No. 10, November 15, 2004, pages 2187-2194. Available at http://www.ncbi.nlm.nih.gov/pubmed/15382089.

[192] Jeannine K. Giacovelli et al., "Insurance Status Predicts Access to Care and Outcomes of Vascular Disease," *Journal of Vascular Surgery*, Vol. 48, No. 4, October 2008, pages 905-911. Available at http://www.ncbi.nlm.nih.gov/pmc/ articles/PMC2582051/?tool=pubmed.

[193] Amy Finkelstein, Sarah Taubman, Bill Wright, Mira Bernstein, Jonathan Gruber, Joseph P. Newhouse, Heidi Allen, Katherine Baicker, and the Oregon Health Study Group, "The Oregon Health Insurance Experiment: Evidence from the First Year," *Quarterly Journal of Economics*, Vol. 127, Issue 3. August 2012. Available at http://www.org/oregon/.

[194] Katherine Baicker and the Oregon Health Study Group, "The Oregon Experiment — Effects of Medicaid on Clinical Outcomes," *New England Journal of Medicine*, Vol. 386, No. 18, May 2, 2013. Available at http://www.nejm.org/doi/full/10.1056/NEJMsa1212321#t=article.

[195] Aaron Carroll and Austin Frakt, "Oregon and Medicaid and Evidence and Chill, People!," *Incidental Economist*, May 1, 2013. Available at http://theincidentaleconomist.com/wordpress/oregon-and-medicaid-and-evidence-and-chill-people/.

[196] Whitney R. Johnson, "The Impact of Health Reform on HSAs," *Benefits Quarterly*, Third Quarter 2011. Available at http://www.ifebp.org/ inforequest/0160537.pdf.

[197] Ibid.

[198] "ObamaCare Flatlines: Tax Man Cometh," Conference Blog, GOP. gov, April 6, 2010. Available at http://www.gop.gov/blog/10/04/06/ObamaCare-flatlines-tax-man-cometh.

[199] "Young Adults and the Affordable Care Act: Protecting Young Adults and Eliminating Burdens on Businesses and Families," U.S. Department of Labor. Available at http://www.dol.gov/ebsa/pdf/faq-dependentcoverage.pdf.

[200] "The WellPoint Revelation: Private insurance premiums could triple under ObamaCare," *Wall Street Journal*, October 28, 2009. Available at http://online.wsj.com/article/SB10001424052748703567204574499034177212064.html.

[201] "Health Care Reform Premium Impact in Ohio — December 2009 Addendum," *WellPoint*, December 2009. Available at http://www.wellpoint.com/prodcontrib/groups/wellpoint/@wp_news_research/documents/wlp_assets/pw_d014994.pdf.

[202] Mark V. Pauly, *Health Benefits at Work: An Economic and Political Analysis of Employment-based Health Insurance* (Ann Arbor: University of Michigan Press, 1997). Also see David Cutler, "Public Policy for Health Care," in Alan Auerbach, ed., *Fiscal Policy: Lessons from Economic Research* (Cambridge: MIT Press, 1997), pages 59-98.

[203] John C. Goodman, "The Cruel Things Obama Is Doing To The Labor Market," *Forbes*, May 27, 2013. Available at http://www.forbes.com/sites/johngoodman/2013/05/10/the-cruel-things-obama-is-doingto-the-labor-market/.

[204] Samantha Maziarz Christmann, "Wegmans cuts health benefits for part-time workers," *Buffalo News*, July 11, 2013. Available at http://www.buffalonews.com/apps/pbcs.dll/article?AID=/20130710/BUSINESS/130719892/1003.

[205] John C. Goodman, "The Cruel Things Obama Is Doing To The Labor Market." Also see Chad Terhune, "Part-timers to lose pay amid health act's new math," *Los Angeles Times*, May 2, 2013. Available at http://articles.latimes.com/2013/may/02/business/la-fi-part-time-healthcare-20130502.

[206] "Electronic Code Of Federal Regulations, Part 4-Labor Standards For Federal Service Contracts," United States Government printing office, Title 29 Labor, December 30, 2013. Available at http://www.ecfr.gov/cgi-bin/text-idx?rgn=div5&node=29:1.1.1.1.5.

[207] Paul Christiansen, "To Outsmart ObamaCare, Go Protean," *Wall Street Journal*, January 23, 2013, available at http://online.wsj.com/news/articles/SB10001424127887324461604578193472562389926.

[208] Robert Pear, "Some Employers Could Opt Out of Insurance Market, Raising Others' Costs," *New York Times*, February 17, 2013. Available at http://www.nytimes.com/2013/02/18/us/allure-of-self-insurance-draws-concern-over-costs.html.

[209] Timothy Jost, "Implementing Health Reform: Grandfathered Plans," *Health Affairs* blog, June 15th, 2010. Available at http://healthaffairs.org/blog/2010/06/15/implementing-health-reform-grandfathered-plans/.

[210] Ricardo Alonso-Zaldivar, "Like Your Health Care Policy? You May Be Losing It," Associated Press, May 29, 2013. Available at http://bigstory.ap.org/article/your-health-care-policy-you-may-be-losing-it.

[211] "Interim Final Rules for Group Health Plans and Health Insurance Coverage Relating to Status as a Grandfathered Health Plan under the Patient Protection and Affordable Care," U.S. Department of Health and Human Services, July 2010, page 54. Available at http://www.ncpa.org/pdfs/employees-not-grandfathered-in.pdf#page=54.

[212] Ibid.

[213] Chris Jacobs, "Did Unions Just Obtain Another Backroom Health Care Deal?" Republican Policy Committee, June 14, 2010. Available at http://www.ncpa.org/pdfs/E-mail_from_Chris_Jacobs_RPC_061510.pdf.

[214] Robert Pear, "Small Firms' Offer of Plan Choices Under Health Law Delayed," *New York Times*, April 1, 2013. Available at http://www.nytimes.com/2013/04/02/us/politics/option-for-small-business-health-plan-delayed.html.

[215] Dan Danner, "ObamaCare vs. Small Business," *Wall Street Journal*, May 27, 2010. Available at http://online.wsj.com/article/SB10001424052748704113504575264802756326086.html.

[216] Richard V. Burkhauser, Sean Lyons and Kosali I. Simon, "The Importance of the Meaning and Measurement of "Affordable" in the Affordable Care Act," National Bureau of Economic Research, Working Paper No. 17279, August 2011. Available at http://www.NBER.org/papers/w17279.

[217] "White House Unveils Subsidies To Preserve Early-Retiree Coverage," *Kaiser Health News*, May 5, 2010. Available at http://www.kaiserhealthnews.org/Daily-Reports/2010/May/05/early-retirees-wednes.aspx.

[218] John C. Goodman, "ObamaCare Slams Employers, Retirees."

[219] Board of Trustees, "2010 Annual Report of The Boards of Trustees of The Federal Hospital Insurance and Federal Supplementary Medical Insurance Trust Funds," Federal Hospital Insurance And Federal Supplementary Medical Insurance Trust Funds, Table IV.B8.— Part D Enrollment. Available at http://www.cms.gov/ReportsTrustFunds/downloads/tr2010.pdf.

[220] Monica Davey and Abby Goodnough, "Detroit Looks to Health Law to Ease Costs," *New York Times*, July 28, 2013. Available at http://www.nytimes.com/2013/07/29/us/detroit-looks-to-health-law-to-ease-costs.html.

[221] Bruce Japsen, "ObamaCare's 73% Medicaid Pay Raise For Doctors Is Delayed," Forbes Pharma & Healthcare blog, March 15, 2013. Available at http://www.forbes.com/sites/brucejapsen/2013/03/15/ObamaCares-73-medicaid-pay-raise-for-doctors-is-delayed/.

[222] Medicare Payments to Physicians (Updated), *Health Affairs*, Health Policy Briefs, January 10, 2013. Available at http://www.healthaffairs.org/healthpolicybriefs/brief.php?brief_id=83.

[223] Joseph P. Newhouse, "Assessing Health Reform's Impact On Four Key Groups Of Americans."

[224] Carolyn Needham and Irene Switzer, "Medicare's New Price Control Board," National Center for Policy Analysis, Brief Analysis No. 771, September 11, 2012. Available at http://www.ncpa.org/pdfs/ba771.pdf.

[225] Jason R. Barro, Robert S. Huckman and Daniel P. Kessler, "The effects of cardiac specialty hospitals on the cost and quality of medical care," *Journal of Health Economics*, Vol. 25, December 6, 2005, pages 702-721. Availableathttp://www.hbs.edu/healthcare/pdf/barro_huckman_kessler.pdf.

[226] John C. Goodman, "How ObamaCare Is Affecting the Practice of Medicine," John Goodman's Health Policy Blog, July 3, 2013. Available at http://healthblog.ncpa.org/how-ObamaCare-is-affecting-the-practice-of-medicine-2/.

[227] Scott Gottlieb, "The Doctor Won't See You Now. He's Clocked Out."

[228] "Retail medical clinics: From Foe to Friend?" Accenture, June 2013. Available at http://www.accenture.com/SiteCollectionDocuments/PDF/Accenture-Retail-Medical-Clinics-From-Foe-to-Friend.pdf.

About the National Center for Policy Analysis

The National Center for Policy Analysis (NCPA) is a 501(c)(3) nonprofit, nonpartisan public policy research organization that was established in 1983. The NCPA's mission is to develop and promote private alternatives to government regulation and control, solving problems by relying on the strength of the competitive, entrepreneurial private sector. The organization primarily focuses on topics such as health care reform, taxes, retirement, the economy and environmental regulation.

The NCPA's motto is *Ideas Changing The World*, which reflects the belief that ideas have a tremendous ability to change the course of human events. The NCPA plays an active role in utilizing that ability to establish positive change by identifying, encouraging and aggressively communicating the best scholarly research. By producing credible, accurate and timely analyses of public policy options, the NCPA is increasingly providing leadership to the entire nation and helping to shape the policy agenda of today and the future.

Working with scholars at colleges, universities and other think tanks, the NCPA examines issues that have a significant impact on the lives of all Americans, proposing innovative, market-driven solutions. For instance, the NCPA is widely recognized for developing the concept of Health Savings Accounts (HSAs). In 2003, Congress and the president made HSAs available to all Americans, potentially revolutionizing the entire health care industry. More than 30 million people now control some of their own health care dollars through HSAs or similar accounts.

The NCPA shares its solutions with policy makers, journalists, business and community leaders and the general public.